THE SOCIAL CONTEXT OF COGNITIVE DEVELOPMENT

The Guilford Series on Social and Emotional Development

CLAIRE B. KOPP and STEVEN R. ASHER, *Editors*

Children and Marital Conflict:
The Impact of Family Dispute and Resolution
E. Mark Cummings and Patrick Davies

Emotional Development in Young Children
Susanne A. Denham

The Development of Emotional Competence
Carolyn Saarni

The Social Context of Cognitive Development
Mary Gauvain

The Social Context of Cognitive Development

Mary Gauvain

Foreword by Robert S. Siegler

gp

THE GUILFORD PRESS
New York   London

© 2001 The Guilford Press
A Division of Guilford Publications, Inc.
72 Spring Street, New York, NY 10012
www.guilford.com

Printed in the United States of America

This book is printed on acid-free paper.

Last digit is print number: 9 8 7 6 5 4 3

Library of Congress Cataloging-in-Publication Data

Gauvain, Mary
   The social context of cognitive development / by Mary Gauvain.
      p.   cm. — (The Guilford series on social and emotional
   development)
   Includes bibliographical references and index.
   ISBN 1-57230-516-9 (hc.) — ISBN 1-57230-610-6 (pbk.)
   1. Cognition in children—Social aspects. 2. Cognition and culture.
I. Title. II. Series.

BF723.C5 G38 2000
155.4′13—dc21

                                                                00-062259

*To my husband, Jim, and
our children, Benjamin and Graeme*

About the Author

Mary Gauvain, PhD, is Professor of Psychology at the University of California at Riverside. She received her master's degree in Sociology of Education from Stanford University and her doctoral degree in Developmental Psychology from the University of Utah. She is a fellow of the American Psychological Association and has served on the Executive Committee of the APA Division of Developmental Psychology. She is also a member of the Society for Research in Child Development. Her research on children's cognitive development in social and cultural contexts is widely published and has been funded by the National Institute of Child Health and Human Development and The Spencer Foundation, among others.

Foreword

Among the greatest differences between human beings and other animals is the range of mechanisms through which we learn. Like other species, people learn through association, habituation, and operant and classical conditioning. Unlike other species, people also learn a great deal through conversation, intentional teaching, and use of cultural artifacts such as books and number systems.

Although learning continues throughout life, childhood is the time in which it is most dramatic. Indeed, the importance of learning, relative to performance, is central to our definition of childhood. Infants, toddlers, and preschoolers are constantly acquiring new capabilities; rapid learning of a broad range of skills is essential for normal development. On the other hand, how well they perform a given task ordinarily is unimportant. The quality of the pictures they draw, their skill at playing games, and their knowledge of songs and television characters matters little. What is important is that they, and school-age children as well, learn to act in ways that will allow them to perform effectively in future settings. In contrast, adults' performance is frequently very important. How well they do at work, at driving a car, and at parenting matters a great deal to their well-being and to that of those around them. Five hundred years ago, 14-year-olds were adults, because they had learned enough that they could function as adults; today, they are children, because they need to learn so much more before they can function in adult capacities.

Despite the obvious importance of learning in children's lives, the dominant theories of cognitive development over the past 40 years have paid surprisingly little attention to it. This is true of Piagetian, information processing, and theory-theory approaches alike. Each of these has focused most intensely on how children think at different ages rather than on how they acquire those ways of thinking. In part, this is because it makes sense to describe what children know at different points in development before trying to explain how they get from here to there. This is partly a reaction to the weaknesses of older learning theory approaches to development, and reflects partially the pragmatic realization that it is easier to describe what children know than how they acquire new knowledge. All of these factors have conspired to limit current understanding of change processes in children's thinking and to create depictions of children that are at odds with everyday observation of their dynamism.

In *The Social Context of Cognitive Development*, Mary Gauvain has identified the problems that have arisen through inadequate attention to learning and has set out to address them. The book is unique among those I have read in its depth of integration of insights from sociocultural and information-processing approaches. Gauvain makes a compelling case that the two approaches are complementary, with each providing important insights about children's learning that are missing from the other.

As Gauvain notes, to the extent that information-processing approaches have examined learning, they have focused on mechanisms that operate during the course of particular learning episodes. These mechanisms include encoding new features of the task, identifying rules that consistently solve the problems being presented, drawing analogies between the new situation and previous ones, choosing among alternative strategies, and so on. Precise assessment of knowledge, both before and after the learning episode, has also been emphasized. On the other hand, information-processing analyses have had little to say about how children learn through interactions with their parents and other knowledgeable individuals, how children learn through interactions with peers of roughly equal knowledge, and how the culture within which children develop influences the skills, knowledge, and values that they acquire. In short, information-processing approaches have focused on the internal cognitive processes involved in learning to the exclusion of social processes that are also involved in most learning.

As Gauvain also notes, sociocultural approaches to cognitive development have strengths and weaknesses complementary to those of information-processing approaches. Sociocultural approaches have focused on the way in which parents, teachers, other adults, siblings, and peers influence children's development. They also have emphasized how learning is influenced by relationship variables, such as attachment status, previous interactions, and friendships. Conversely, sociocultural approaches have had little to say about the precise cognitive processes through which children internalize the lessons learned in social contexts, and have emphasized events during the learning episode more than precise analyses of what was learned. Although children's contributions to their own learning are acknowledged at a theoretical level, empirical research within this tradition has focused on how other people and cultural practices shape learning.

A major argument within this book is that the operation of the social context is just as significant a learning mechanism (or set of learning mechanisms) as the types of mechanisms emphasized by information-processing approaches. Gauvain notes that social processes greatly influence both what is learned and how the learning occurs. As she states,

> Involvement with others, either at play or at work, creates opportunities for individuals to evaluate and refine their understanding as they are exposed to the thinking of others and as they participate in creating shared understanding. In this way, social experience can serve as a mechanism for developmental change. (p. 40)

This strikes me as an important observation. At minimum, it challenges information-processing theorists to account for the effects of social interaction on learning. Most likely, any attempt to meet this challenge will require expanding the types of cognitive processes that have been considered in information-processing accounts of learning. To cite just one such challenge: Explain why securely attached children learn more than insecurely attached children when engaged in joint problem solving with their mothers. It seems unlikely that this and other phenomena demonstrated by sociocultural researchers can be explained completely in terms of encoding, associate competition, rule formation, strategy choice, and so on.

Gauvain also makes a strong case that considering the social context is crucial for understanding the types of learning mechanisms that have been proposed by those who take an information-processing approach. For example, she notes that children's strategy choices reflect not only their own cognitive processes but also the support of other, more knowledgeable, people. Adults, in particular, teach children new strategies for obtaining goals, guide their attention to useful strategies that they have learned previously, help them execute approaches that they could not execute by themselves, and inform them about which choices are most highly valued in their community.

To support her theoretical position, Gauvain reviews a wide range of research on four topics: attention, memory, problem solving, and planning. Her review focuses on learning that occurs through interactions with family members, peers, and other people and on situations that occur frequently in everyday life: toddlers looking to their mother to observe her reaction to an unfamiliar object; parents and children planning trips to the grocery store, assembling puzzles, and discussing experiences that occurred at birthday parties, school, and play; children asking for explanations of everyday phenomena such as where rain comes from, and so on. Bringing together in a single place this rich and varied set of findings on children's learning in the social context constitutes a major contribution in and of itself.

For those not yet convinced that the field of cognitive development needs to emphasize learning to a greater extent than it has in the past, this book makes a compelling case that the field should move in this direction. For those of us who are already convinced of this point, the book makes an equally compelling case that understanding children's learning will require combining insights from sociocultural and information-processing analyses as well as insights still to come.

ROBERT S. SIEGLER
Carnegie Mellon University

Preface

*I*n the 1970s a revolution in the study of cognitive development began to brew. As is the case in all revolutions, this one started relatively quietly and grew with time. It emerged at a precipitous time for the field. Disenchantment with Piagetian approaches was on the rise. Innovative ideas from neighboring disciplines that were not really developmental in approach, such as information processing and cognitive science, were attracting much interest. However, the revolution to which I refer was not concerned with either of these trajectories. Rather, it was struggling with an entirely different set of ideas. Some of these ideas appeared in the writings and observations of developmental psychologists based on their research in non-Western communities. The book *The Cultural Context of Learning and Thinking*, by Cole, Gay, Glick, and Sharp, published in 1971, is a landmark contribution along these lines. Other related ideas came from the writings of Vygotsky, which were introduced in English translation in the 1960s and 1970s. The influential *Thought and Language* appeared in 1962 and *Mind in Society* in 1978.

At the heart of this revolution was increasing uncertainty and discomfort with views of development that ignored the context of cognitive growth and intelligent performance. Research was making it clear that the context of behavior, especially the social and cultural context, was critical to defining what people did, what they learned, and how they developed this understanding. The researchers raising these questions referred to context in a variety of ways—as culture, social context, situation, and activity setting, to name a few. But the overall message was the same. Perspectives that concentrate on internal processes of cognitive development and ignore external processes and the interaction of the two are simply unable to provide a complete account of the emergence of the human intellect. For some, this may have seemed like a methodological critique, one that had been made many times before in discussions about demand characteristics. But it was not a methodological critique at all; it was a theoretical and metatheoretical critique.

Like all revolutions, this "change of mind" took time. Over time there have been many participants, some false starts, and some monumental insights. Now, a generation later, it is impossible to pick up a developmental psychology text that does not include some discussion of the social context of cognitive development. So, in some measure, the revolution has been a success. However, in most instances, with a few notable exceptions (see, e.g., Cole & Cole, 1996), the social context of cognitive development is relegated to a secondary role to research that concentrates on individual, internal changes unconcerned with social factors. In my view, this too will change and the social nature of cognitive development will be increasingly incorporated as a defining characteristic of human intelligence and its development.

In the meantime, there is still much work to be done. Critical to moving this perspective forward is examination of what has been learned to date about cognitive development from a social vantage point. This is the topic of this book. This book does not pretend to provide an inclusive treatment of all areas of cognitive development from a social-contextual perspective. Nor does it even cover all areas of cognitive development. Rather, its aim is to explain and explore this approach by examining research in several of the primary domains of cognitive development with one question in mind: Has this perspective advanced understanding of cognitive development in each of these domains, and if so, how?

In order to answer this question, it is necessary to explain a sociocultural perspective in some detail. Although the book does not address many of the complex theoretical and philosophical issues raised by scholars in a variety of disciplines, including literary criticism, semiotics, and history, about this approach, it does cover the basic premises that underlie current developmental research based on this perspective. The main questions of the book are rather straightforward; they are, in fact, the same questions that might be addressed in any book on cognitive development: How do we learn to think and why do we end up thinking the way we do?

AN OVERVIEW OF THE BOOK

To answer these questions, this book discusses recent theory and research on the social context of cognitive development. It takes the view that the social settings in which children live and grow provide both opportunities and constraints for cognitive development. A central purpose of this book is to convey the utility of a social-contextual perspective to the study of cognitive development and not merely criticize traditional avenues of investigation.

In Part I of the book, the basic formulation of a social approach to cognitive development is described. Chapter 1 is a general introduction to this approach, illustrated with examples from the memoirs of notable people. These examples are included to highlight the fact that even though psychologists may have overlooked the social contribution to cognitive development, this contribution has not been bypassed by other keen observers of the human condition when they recount their own upbringing.

The introduction is followed by several chapters that address some of the critical questions that underlie an inquiry into the social nature of cognitive development, including how cognitive changes occur. To address this question, Chapter 2 focuses on mechanisms, that is, the "how," of cognitive development, with particular attention to the social processes that support and lead intellectual growth. Chapter 3 examines the social and cultural foundations of cognitive development, and includes discussion of some of the primary agents of cognitive socialization.

Part II concentrates on what can be learned about certain specific domains of cognitive development when social context is taken into account. Four domains are examined: attention (Chapter 4), memory (Chapter 5), problem solving (Chapter 6), and planning (Chapter 7). The concluding chapter, Chapter 8, revisits the question of whether and how social context can be conceptualized as a mechanism of cognitive change. It examines the theoretical and practical utility of this approach and speculates about why its impact on the field has, to date, been rather limited. Finally, in the hope of advancing the study of cognitive development through the use of this perspective, future directions of research are proposed.

Acknowledgments

*N*o scholarly book is written without the guidance and support of others. I was fortunate to have two graduate advisors, Barbara Rogoff and Irv Altman, who taught me in immeasurable ways about the connection between context and human development. To both of them I am truly grateful. The writing of this book was greatly aided by the comments and suggestions of the editor, Claire Kopp, to whom I am most thankful. Finally, I thank my husband, Jim Hoste, for his patience, support, and constant interest in my work and my life, and our children, Benjamin and Graeme, for teaching me firsthand about the progress and pitfalls of cognitive development.

Contents

THE SOCIAL CONTEXT OF COGNITIVE DEVELOPMENT

❧ PART I

THE SOCIAL FOUNDATIONS
OF COGNITIVE DEVELOPMENT

Chapter 1

Introduction

Four-year-old Graeme spies his mother at the kitchen counter beginning to make a cake. He walks to the table opposite the counter, grabs hold of a chair, carries it to the counter, sets it next to his mother, and steps onto the chair. He asks, "What are we making?" Then he takes hold of the bowl and a wooden spoon and eyes the ingredients. Meanwhile, his mother, who had previously arranged the ingredients, the utensils, and the recipe on the counter, has started to measure the flour.

This interaction is typical of the types of social situations young children experience everyday throughout the world. A child and a more experienced partner work together to accomplish a practical, meaningful goal—in this case, making a cake. What happened after the child immersed himself in the activity? Because this is an experience I shared with one of my sons, I can assure you that the cake did, eventually, get made. This activity, of course, did not unfold in the same way that I had planned. Rather than making the cake on my own, I made it in collaboration with my child. Collaboration involved adjustments on both ends, as I made the process understandable and accessible to my son and he made his understanding and needs known to me.

Interactions such as this offer children the opportunity to develop many important skills and convey rich socioemotional, cognitive, and cultural messages. Both partners change over the course of the experience. The child learns about the activity and how to accomplish the goal. The adult changes her behavior as she adapts to the child's needs.

3

For instance, the adult slows down the activity, as when she provides the child with adequate time to add the ingredients to the bowl—something she would ordinarily do much more quickly. She also modifies certain aspects of the task to support the child's participation. For example, measuring the ingredients proceeds more carefully and overtly than when she works alone. As an adult and a child work together, they learn about each other's needs, how to help and support one another, and how to enjoy each other's company. They also learn about each other as individuals, such as what the child or adult enjoys about the activity or what parts are easy or difficult for one or for both of them. Whereas the child may become frustrated measuring the ingredients, the mother may become frustrated stirring the thick batter. In cultural terms, a number of conventions that are valued in the community in which the mother and child live are part of the interaction. Conventions of social interaction itself, such as how to ask and answer questions and how to explain ideas, organize much of the flow of the exchange. Other cultural features are embedded in the activity in the form of the measurement conventions used, the fact that precise measurement is important, and the idea that people make special foods for certain reasons.

This book is concerned with everyday interactions like the one I described because of the important role they play as contexts for cognitive development. Experiences such as these provide children with the opportunity to observe and participate in more skilled performances than they can accomplish on their own, and this may lead directly to learning and development. The activity of cooking, for instance, entails many discrete, easily observable behaviors that can be identified with an understandable and desired goal. This provides the child with the opportunity to connect certain means–ends relations, a type of understanding that is foundational to causal reasoning. The child may receive instruction from the mother as she tells him what to do in order to help. Such didactic instruction is a mainstay of adult–child interaction, especially in certain learning contexts and cultural communities. The mother may also structure the task in ways that make working with the materials, and thereby learning how to reach the goal, more accessible for the child. For example, she may arrange the ingredients or adapt the activities to mesh with the child's skills. Or she may coordinate her actions with those of the child to support his participation in activities that are still too difficult for him to do on his own. For instance, she may hold the bowl as the child stirs the batter. The mother may also perform some actions so that the child can readily observe them, and thereby serve as models for behavior.

Social–cognitive transactions such as this are ubiquitous. They emerge spontaneously and frequently in the course of daily life. They typically appear during practical, routine activities, and as a result are often understandable to children and have a high probability of occurrence. They are the types of activities for which children in a household are ordinarily present and they are often directed toward a goal of importance to the child. Not surprisingly, many of these instances involve behavioral routines and practices related to protection, warmth, and nutrition, such as opening or closing windows, laundering clothes, or preparing food. The fact that these activities are often conducted by a person or persons of much importance or interest to the child also facilitates learning.

Due to their frequency of occurrence and their inherent attraction and importance to children, social situations such as these compose the bedrock experiences through which children live and learn in everyday life. One key question for developmental psychology is the following: What are the consequences of social experiences such as these for human intellectual development? To address this question, in this book I examine the social context of cognitive development. My particular interest is how the social world organizes and directs intellectual growth. I concentrate on psychological theory and research on this topic; however, I also draw on the observations of anthropologists and the writings of literary and public figures. All this evidence is used to support the claims that social experience is an essential component of cognitive development, that social influences on intellectual development permeate most aspects of young children's lives, and that lack of attention to this contribution presents serious limitations to the study of intellectual growth. These claims do not imply that all the details of this story are completely understood or that even all the important questions on this topic have yet been raised. They simply suggest that the long-held approach of dividing the intellectual from the social and, by extension, the emotional parts of growth has kept us from understanding key components of cognitive development.

THE SOCIAL FOUNDATION OF THE MIND

One of our most amazing qualities as human beings is our ability to think. Humans think in all sorts of ways and about all sorts of things. Sometimes our thinking is complex and awe-inspiring. At other times it is simple and practical. Yet even in the course of everyday, run-of-the-mill, practical thinking, the capabilities of the human mind are truly impressive.

The basic neural structure that supports the human intellect is present at birth. However, the many capabilities of the mind that we rely on in our everyday functioning as adults emerge over a fairly long period of time. In fact, our species, *Homo sapiens sapiens,* has the longest period of physical dependency by the young on mature members of the group of any species on the planet. This lengthy period provides protection for the young, along with warmth and food—all of which are critical to survival. It is also sufficiently long to support the extensive process of social, emotional, and intellectual learning that prepares children for mature participation in their community.

Scientists who study human development have tended to study the intellectual, social, and emotional aspects of development separately, concentrating on one of these areas of growth. This decision has more to do with the nature of science, the divide-and-conquer (or reductionist) approach to the study of complex systems, than it does with the nature of human development itself. This scientific approach can obscure the fact that these three aspects of human development—the social, the emotional, and the cognitive—are interdependent and seamlessly intertwined. Over time they define and refine the course of growth, and together they describe the landscape of human development. Although, as I have stated, this point is not always evident in scientific research, it is exceedingly clear when development is considered from the vantage point of the organism rather than that of the scientist.

For the organism, who must develop and function as a unified social–emotional–intellectual whole, the interrelation of these three aspects of development is crucial to everyday activity. This does not mean that in any particular circumstance one or another of these aspects may not dominate. At any given point in time, a person may be involved in an activity that is predominantly intellectual or predominantly emotional or predominantly social. But even in such instances, the other two aspects of human functioning are present to some degree. Consider the master chess player competing in a tournament. He or she is unquestionably engaged in an intellectual activity as he or she deliberates over strategies and plans moves. However, the master's intense concentration and deliberate actions are supported by emotions such as heightened arousal, a desire to win, joy in playing, and so forth. The social dimension is apparent in the competition, most obviously in the moves of the opponent. But it is also evident in the nature and conventions of the game itself. Violations of these conventions would disqualify the player. From a historical perspective, the opponents' actions reflect the society and culture in which the game was developed and also that in which the player learned to play.

My primary aim in this book is to bring the social and emotional contributions to intellectual growth more clearly into view. There has been a tendency to study cognitive development with little attention to social and emotional contributions, what Brown, Bransford, Ferrara, and Campione (1983) referred to as the "cold cognition" approach. However, the separation of the cognitive, emotional, and social facets of human development introduces serious problems to the study of mental growth. Although the observation and assessment of children's independent cognitive performances in laboratory conditions provide control for examining certain influences on behavior, this approach ignores a fundamental characteristic of human intellectual development. Children develop thinking skills while in the company of other people—typically in the company of people important to them. They are guided in this endeavor by the resources and tools of their community, many of which were devised by prior members of the group, and therefore stem from and represent the child's social and cultural world. This book concentrates on the social and emotional context of intellectual development, however, along the way it does attend to the cultural context of development. Although a complete examination of the cultural context of human development is beyond the scope of this book, some discussion of culture and development is necessary to any study of cognitive development concerned with the social, material, and symbolic components of intelligent action and its development. Because most higher level cognitive functions draw on these components in some way, culture contributes in a critical and pervasive manner to the shape of cognitive development.

In addition to identifying the role of social, emotional, and cultural experience in cognitive development, there is a need to clarify the linkage between a social or contextual approach to cognitive development and more traditional approaches that have tended to concentrate on the internal mechanisms of development and to ignore the external contributions to this process. In order to reach the goal of a more integrated developmental psychology, it is especially important to describe the contributions of social, emotional, and cultural experience to cognitive development in a way that reconciles observations of children's intellectual performances in controlled, often solitary, laboratory conditions with those obtained in more naturalistic settings. Although the solitary laboratory context may be an unusual context for children relative to their daily experiences, it is nonetheless a context within which children are able to display cognitive skills. Thus, the integration of laboratory and nonlaboratory observations is critical to cognitive developmental theory. Not only will such integration advance theory, it will also serve more practical goals. In particular, it may clarify how information obtained via laboratory observations relates to children's thinking in the everyday settings in which they live and grow.

An important question that arises from this inquiry is whether social experience is a necessary and sufficient condition for cognitive growth. It is clearly not a sufficient condition. The human biological system is an essential co-contributor to this process. However, it does appear that it is a necessary condition, although, from a scientific standpoint, this is said with trepidation. This is because this conjecture is impossible to prove in that human beings do not develop normal intellectual capabilities outside of human social communities. Thus, there are no counterexamples to be found nor any valid (or ethical) experiments that can be conducted on this question. The small bit of evidence that exists regarding the intellectual development of individuals who, due to unfortuitous circumstances, developed as nonsocially as one can imagine for a human being, is consistent with this claim, however. For instance, neither the Wild Boy of Aveyron (Itard, 1801/ 1982), who was abandoned as a child and grew up alone in the forests of France, or Genie (Curtiss, 1977), a severely abused girl reared by her parents in a closet, developed normal intelligence. In one or both of these cases, the child may have had a chromosomal or genetic abnormality from the outset; this is difficult to discount for certain. But the point remains that the prognosis for intellectual development for children reared outside the human social community is extremely bleak.

Although such evidence is suggestive, it cannot, in and of itself, satisfy the question of the essential contribution of social experience to intellectual growth. Another analytical tact is needed. An alternative approach, the one adopted in this book, involves delineating the aspects of human cognitive development that can be better understood when the social context of development is included in the analysis. Much of this book relies on psychological theory and empirical research to examine this question. Another, very different source of information about child development in social context comes in the form of autobiographical accounts. Excerpts from such accounts are used below as an introduction to my discussion of the social context of cognitive development.

REMEMBERING CHILDHOOD

Remembering prior experiences is a common and uniquely human experience (Tulving, 1983). People are not only capable of thinking about the past, they are also able to reflect upon these memories, which may, in turn, lead to a new or different understanding of the self, other people, or the memory itself. Memories of past events are called *episodic memories* in that they recount in some fashion something that happened at a specific time and place. One type of episodic memory, called *auto-biographical memory*, is concerned with specific life events pertaining to the self.

Autobiographical memory emerges in the early years of life, when a child is about 2½ years old, and it develops substantially over the pre-school years (Nelson, 1993). Such memories are linked in both process and content to the social experiences that children have. During social interaction, children learn what to remember, how to formulate their memories, and how to retain them in retrievable or recountable form (Engel, 1995; Fivush, 1988; Hudson, 1990). This does not mean that the events that are remembered were always shared with others when they occurred. Rather, by talking about current and past experiences, children have the opportunity to rehearse these memories and, in so doing, they learn some very important things about the memory itself and the whole process of remembering. For instance, during social re-membering children learn about the conventional narrative form for recounting memories, as well as the types of events and interpretations of events that are of interest or of importance to others. Here is how my son Benjamin, at 5 years of age, explained an incident to his teacher that involved a bloody, but ultimately minor, cut to the head of his 2½-year-old brother, Graeme:

TEACHER: What did you do over the holidays?

BEN: There was an accident.

TEACHER: Oh, what happened?

BEN: My brother jumped on the bed and cut his head on the table. And then, after he cut his head, then the paramedics came and two fire trucks and an ambulance.

TEACHER: Oh, how awful! Then what happened?

BEN: Mommy went with him in the ambulance. I stayed at home with Nana.

In this example, an adult, the child's teacher, used cues to elicit de-tails; she defined an emotional context (not inconsequentially, one con-sistent with the emotional context generated at the time of the event by Ben's family members); and she "steered" the child as he recounted the story. The child used the occasion to describe the aspects of the event that were important and understandable to him. He used a narrative form, an account of an event that is temporally sequenced and conveys meaning. In this narrative, he described the event, as well as information about himself, his family, and his own experience during the event.

Even though what Ben said is very brief, it is clear that this was an emotionally arousing experience for him. Even a short narrative may have deep meaning or value for children (Engel, 1995). This value is enhanced because autobiographical memories are personal in a very interesting way. They help define an individual's own history, and thereby define key features of the self. However, because of the social contributions to autobiographical memory, this history is shaped by the social and cultural world in which development occurs. For instance, autobiographical memories that are considered interesting or that represent valued activities in a particular community are more likely to be elicited by others. If a topic is prohibited or considered distasteful or uninteresting, a memory of such an event is less likely to be told to others, and is therefore less likely to be organized in narrative form or rehearsed through retelling. Even the interpretations of others regarding an event may become part of the autobiographical memory if the retelling triggers a certain response. For instance, if a child describes an experience that adults find amusing, the event may then be remembered not only in terms of the actions and the sequences of these actions, but also in terms of its effect upon others. Since the effect in this example was pleasurable in that it garnered adult interest and attention, it may increase the likelihood of Ben's retelling and therefore remembering the event.

In order to illustrate how cognitive development is affected by social experience, I will describe several examples from autobiographical accounts. Although such accounts are, by their very nature, subjective, they nevertheless tell the story of how an individual integrated the many threads of his or her life into a meaningful, personal whole. Thus, such accounts do not simply describe the events of the person's life, they convey something about the process of development that the person experienced from the person's own perspective. These are useful to present at the outset of this book because they characterize the types of developmental experiences that I believe are central to cognitive growth but are difficult to understand from within the confines of conventional approaches to development that emphasize internal change independent of the social and cultural forces that are integral to the process of intellectual development.

Learning to Think in Social Context

The purpose of a memoir is to convey the passage and sense of a life and not trace the process of cognitive development. As a result, these examples provide mere glimpses into the social context of cognitive development. Later in the book, more systematic research efforts to understand this process are the focus. But as an introduction to the topic, these examples illustrate one theme of this book, namely, the active and varied efforts that parents and others make to support, organize, and direct children's intellectual growth. These efforts include arranging for specific learning activities to occur, regulating the child's participation in activities in which learning occurs, determining the pattern and frequency of routine activities that provide support and direction for emerging cognitive skills, emphasizing activities that encourage learning of valued cultural practices, and modeling strategic behaviors (Cole & Cole, 1996).

Arranging for Specific Learning Activities to Occur

In some cases memoirs explain how parents helped arrange activities for their children that led to the development of a set of behaviors or a way of looking at the world that an individual developed in childhood and then used throughout his or her life. For example, the anthropologist Margaret Mead (1972) wrote a memoir about her childhood called *Blackberry Winter*. In this book Mead recounts how her parents prided themselves on the informal education they provided for their children in their home. Mead and her siblings learned household chores, such as peeling apples, shining tomatoes, and knitting, and academic subjects like reading, algebra, and botany. Her parents also brought skilled workers, such as woodcarvers, carpenters, and artists, into their home to train the children as if they were apprentices. Mead recalled that in her home no aspects of life, including the most mundane acts, were taken for granted—a theme that recurs in her later anthropological writings. Mead also credited her parents with teaching her the importance of using careful observation to understand people who were different from her; indeed, her parents deliberately arranged activities that made this clear. For instance, when Mead was a young girl, her mother's charitable work exposed the future anthropologist to the newly formed immigrant communities of the northeastern United States—an experience that Mead called her first "field work." Through such experiences, Mead believed her parents taught her by their example and instruction and through her participation that the ways in which people live are meaningful and sensible in their own context. This, she claims, led her to the realization that there are many valid ways of living out a life and that the description of these different ways can be interesting and enlightening.

Eleanor Roosevelt (1937) grew up around the same time and in the same region of the United States as Margaret Mead. However, the goals that Roosevelt's parents had for their children led them to arrange very different types of activities in and around the home. Roosevelt described the joys and difficulties of being raised "to do one's duty" as a member of a patrician American family. Philanthropic duties and social grace were both taken very seriously. As early as age 6, Roosevelt's father took her on excursions to help those less advantaged, for example, by serving Thanksgiving dinner at a home for needy children. He also introduced her to the world of society, teaching her how to dress for formal dinners, converse with others in social company, and dance. Roosevelt believed that these lessons, both philanthropic and social, guided her through many circumstances of her life.

What is interesting in these two examples is the intentional and goal-directed efforts made by parents to arrange experiences that would foster their children's intellectual development along particular lines. Although these examples contain two different childrearing approaches, the activities that the parents arranged provided opportunities for their children to develop particular cognitive skills and to interact socially in ways that influenced the understanding they developed of themselves and others during these experiences. How children develop and learn through their participation in meaningful, goal-directed activities is the focus of approaches to cognitive development discussed throughout this book, such as guided participation (Rogoff, 1990) and activity theory (Leont'ev, 1981), that concentrate on the connection between cognitive development, participation, and activity structure.

Regulating the Child's Participation in Activities in Which Learning Occurs

Parents and more experienced individuals not only arrange for activities to occur, they also regulate children's actions or participation in these activities (Rogoff, 1998). Some children live out their youth in settings undergoing tremendous social and political change. Yet even in these instances the everyday routines of social life set the stage for cognitive development. Some of these lessons occur during daily household routines, like cooking, and involve instruction through participation in an everyday problem-solving situation. For instance, Nobel laureate Wole Soyinka (1981) described his boyhood before and during World War II against the backdrop of fading colonialism and emerging nationhood as played out in a small town in western Nigeria. Amid the many heartwarming, and sometimes heart-wrenching, episodes of his young life, Soyinka describes how his mother actively involved the children in everyday activities, like cooking: "We were all in the backyard, she was cooking, which meant that the entire household was occupied with running trivial errands for her, holding a spoon or a cup" (p. 70).

This scene is not unlike the one described at the beginning of this chapter and others that occur for children every day in communities throughout the world. These serve as a source of *guided participation* (Rogoff, 1990) in which children learn and practice new skills with the assistance of more experienced others. In time, children show increasing regulation of these activities on their own. For example, the French author Simone de Beauvoir (1959) describes how, when growing up during World War I, she often helped her mother and other relatives fulfill some of the duties that French citizens took on during the war. Her mother taught her how to knit hats for the soldiers and she helped her aunt distribute food to the wounded at the railway station. In a self-regulated extension of these early learning experiences, de Beauvoir took it upon herself to collect and distribute food to an isolated refugee child who joined her class at school.

Determining the Pattern and Frequency of Routine Activities That Provide Support and Direction for Emerging Cognitive Skills

The childhood memoir of the Pulitzer Prize–winning historian Doris Kearns Goodwin (1997) provides an interesting illustration of how her father established a routine, a pattern of behavior, that involved father and child—one that had consequences, according to Goodwin, for her intellectual development. By the time Goodwin was 6 years old she was already, like her father, a huge baseball fan. In the summer of her sixth year, her father decided to teach her how to record baseball scores and statistics about the players during a game. This allowed her to keep track of the games of their beloved home team, the Brooklyn Dodgers, that were played when her father was at work. Goodwin writes that "night after night he taught me the odd collection of symbols, numbers, and letters that enable a baseball lover to record every action of the game" (p. 13). When her father arrived home in the evening, she would recount the game for him, play by play. Goodwin points to a direct link between this activity and her current occupation as a historian. She writes that "these nightly recountings provided me with my first lessons in the narrative art." Her father coached her in this narrative form as he asked her about the game, the players, and the plays. He always started with the general questions, like "How many hits did Jackie Robinson get?" and then moved into the more subtle ones, like "Was the strikeout called or swinging?" By decoding her symbols and boxes, Goodwin could report the entire game to her father. This ritual went on night after night for the entire summer. By the end of the summer, Goodwin says, she was hooked on baseball and on the "telling of a good story." For Goodwin, the systematic and thorough approach that she uses in her histories has a formative link to the comprehensive strategy imparted in this early social-learning experience. This process is akin to that described by Vygotsky (1978) as functioning in the zone of proximal development, a process he considered central to intellectual change. For Vygotsky, learning in the zone of proximal development is a dynamic, interactional process in which both the more and the less experienced partners actively generate understanding and cognitive growth.

Goodwin's father used a direct instructional approach to establish a shared routine activity that steered his daughter's intellectual development along desired lines, and the pace of the baseball season helped regulate the frequency of its occurrence. Other memoirs emphasize the less direct approach that parents often use to provide developmental opportunities by organizing established routines in particular ways. In these instances, opportunities for interaction in the zone of proximal development may easily arise. Benjamin Franklin (1771/1961) recalled how, at the dinner table, his father "liked to have as often as he could, some sensible friend or neighbor to converse with, and always took care to start some ingenious or useful topic for discourse which might tend to improve the minds of his children" (p. 24). Franklin attributed his insatiable lifelong curiosity to this type of routine household experience. He also claimed that one unintended consequence of this was that he developed an indifference to the kind of food that was served for dinner because he considered the conversation, "food of the mind," more important than the actual meal. Unfortunately, Franklin does not detail any dinnertime conversations in a way that gives insight into the types of interactional exchanges that were of interest to Vygotsky in his notion of the zone of proximal development. However, Franklin's comment about his insatiable curiosity implies that he played an active, questioning role in these situations, and suggests that these experiences may have engendered the type of interaction central to operating in the zone of proximal development.

Emphasizing Activities That Encourage the Learning of Valued Cultural Practices

Many of the routine activities that parents engage in with their children contain implicit messages about cultural values pertaining to cognitive skills. Some of these involve passing on to children ways of using tools or artifacts that support mental activity. One of the most well-known and respected memoirs of childhood, *The Diary of Anne Frank* (1952), illustrates this point. This diary, written during the years that Anne hid with her family and friends from the Nazis, is not a memoir in the usual sense. Her tragic death in a concentration camp at age 14 stole from Anne the chance to look back on her youth, as others have, from the vantage point of adulthood. Nevertheless, Anne's words show that even in this extremely harrowing and restrictive circumstance some features of normal family life occurred. Embedded in these experiences were efforts by Anne's parents to teach their children routine behaviors that embodied valued cultural practices. For instance, Anne and her sister continued their studies while they were in hiding, and the adults who were present, especially their father, played an instrumental role in facilitating their learning. On February 27, 1943, Anne wrote: "Daddy has emptied a card index box for Margot and me, and put cards in it. It is to be a book card system, then we can write down which books we have read, who they are by, etc." (p. 79). Here, Mr. Frank teaches his children a filing system. In so doing he provides his children with a material tool, or cultural artifact, to help them record and organize their memory—in this case via a listing of the books they have read. Lists such as this are a specialized way of organizing knowledge. The practice of listing stems from culture, and it exerts important changes on human cognition, including the symbolic representation of ideas and ways of accounting for time (Goody, 1977). Memoirs of childhood often recount instances like this one described by Anne Frank in which parents introduce children to the valued tools of their community that are then used by children to support or extend developing cognitive skill.

Not all cultural messages from parents are related to material artifacts and their use. Some pertain to conventional values and behaviors. These often reflect the aspirations that parents have for their children. For families that emigrate from one community to another, the cultural messages parents convey may be especially clear as old and young members struggle with the challenges of living in two or more cultural worlds simultaneously. In his childhood memoir, the writer Richard Rodriguez (1982) expresses the view that some of the lessons his parents taught him helped him to assimilate European American culture. He describes how after his parents moved to the United States from Mexico, they faced many adjustments. In particular, the upper-class lifestyle the family enjoyed in Mexico was abruptly altered. Yet Rodriguez's parents passed on aspects of their past upper-class life in the behaviors they taught their children, such as certain social graces and manners, and in so doing changed their children's future. He writes that "very early, they taught me the *propria* way of eating *como los ricos*. And I was carefully taught elaborate formulas of polite greeting and parting" (p. 122). For Rodriguez, these skills gave him access to the middle-class lifestyle and goals of the United States, including a university degree and a career as a writer—goals that his parents hoped he would realize.

Modeling Strategic Behaviors

Parents often demonstrate behavioral approaches, or strategies, in front of their children that serve as models for the children's future behaviors. Although much psychological research has focused on the role of modeling in the development of social behavior, there may also be intellectual consequences of these experiences in terms of social cognition, self-knowledge, and strategies for solving problems.

Poet Maya Angelou (1969) wrote a gripping account about growing up as an African American child during the Great Depression in Stamps, Arkansas. Among the striking images that Angelou conveys are descriptions of how the behaviors and words of her mother and grandmother taught her about pride in oneself, an understanding she believes gave her a handle on combating racism. In one instance, modeling a way of interacting with others was a powerful developmental experience. One day when Angelou and her mother were standing in the front yard, a group of unruly and threatening white children came toward the home. Angelou wrote: "I looked to Momma for direction. She did an excellent job of sagging from her waist down, but from the waist up she seemed to be pulling for the top of the oak tree across the road" (p. 30). When the children arrived at the fence, her mother began to hum a spiritual and displayed a dignified, passive refusal to be baited by the children's jabs. Her mother's actions, according to Angelou, taught her how to respond to threats and helped form the basis of the strategy she has used to combat racism throughout her life.

Not all of the information that parents and others pass on to children about intelligent ways of behaving are taught directly to children. As this example suggests, many of these messages are conveyed as children watch how more mature community members solve the problems of everyday life, a process referred to as *legitimate peripheral participation* (Lave & Wenger, 1991). These modeled behaviors provide children with examples of alternative ways of solving problems. Children are witnesses to these behaviors, they pay attention to and remember them, and they are able to produce them later if and when circumstances allow.

A Common Theme of Childhood Memoirs

These various memoirs emerged at different times and describe different communities throughout the world. They present very different childhoods and unique circumstances of growth. Yet, despite this range of experience, commonality exists. Each memoir recounts one or several major events that shaped the individual's life; these include the births and deaths of loved ones and the wonders and horrors of the world. They also contain detailed descriptions of everyday life—descriptions that include the cast of characters and the flow of everyday, ordinary activities and experiences that were the stuff of the individual's learning and development.

Each of these stories suggest that the social patterns of children's everyday lives are strikingly similar in some fundamental ways. Children, even children who grew up to become the remarkable individuals noted above, spend much of their childhood working and playing alongside other people. These examples suggest that what children do with others in the course of routine, everyday life affects their cognitive development profoundly. This is not a surprising conclusion. Human beings, after all, are social animals, and human development is a social process. But it is a conclusion that until recently has been poorly integrated with the understanding and description of human intellectual growth. The writers of these memoirs implicitly knew this linkage, which is my reason for including them here. The job for developmental psychologists is to make this connection more systematic and explicit. To do so, we need to understand how individual cognitive development is woven into the largely social experience of human growth.

CONCLUDING THOUGHTS

To approach cognitive development as a social process, a process coordinated with the biological and maturational capabilities and constraints of the developing child, requires us to modify certain assumptions about what cognitive development is and what the proper study of it entails. As White and Siegel (1984) wrote: "The contexts in which children live are, with minor exceptions, social contexts. . . . To understand cognitive development across time and space requires seeing it deeply embedded in a social world of occasions, formalities, etiquettes, and dramaturgy" (p. 239). The social context of the developing mind provides children with opportunities to develop cognitive skills in ways suited to the circumstances of their lives. In particular, interactions in the family are primary forces in the early years of childhood in steering the course of cognitive development in social context. These experiences reflect both family goals and values and the cultural community in which growth occurs. However, in order to understand cognitive development in social context, it is important to do more than describe this social context. It is also necessary to explain how the social context works to enact change in individual cognitive functioning. This leads us to a discussion of mechanisms of cognitive growth, the topic of the next chapter.

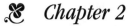

Chapter 2

Processes of Change: The "How" of Cognitive Development

T he years of childhood are marked by tremendous change in what children know and how they think. The activity of knowing, or *cognition,* is a broad topic. It includes basic mental processes like attention, sensation, and perception, as well as higher mental functions like remembering, problem solving, and reasoning. The study of cognitive development investigates how these processes originate and the path they take over the life course. Fundamental to this inquiry are many of the same types of questions that are raised throughout developmental psychology. What capabilities are innate and which ones need to develop? Is development a gradual continuous process or is it characterized by dramatic shifts and discontinuous change? And, finally, how does change occur?

This chapter is concerned with this last question. What processes or mechanisms underlie and direct changes in children's thinking? Given the complexity of the human mental system and the tendency for important areas of development to be multiply determined, there are a number of mechanisms of cognitive change (Siegler, 1989; Sternberg, 1984). This chapter concentrates on one particular mechanism: social experience. In recent years, psychologists and educators have become increasingly interested in the ways in which social experience contributes to thinking and its development. Research indicates that in many areas of cognitive development, but especially in the areas known as *higher mental functions,* the content and process of children's thinking are strongly influenced by social forces. Both the knowledge that children accumulate and the ways that children learn to think about this knowledge are shaped by the social context in which growth occurs.

This chapter begins with a discussion of the mechanisms of cognitive development. This discussion includes the criteria that a process needs to satisfy in order to be considered a mechanism of change. Because social experiences are, in part, external to the organism, this discussion is followed by a brief account of other types of external influences that are considered instrumental to the development of thinking in contemporary theories of cognitive development. The purpose of this discussion is not to discount the contribution of any particular set of external influences that have been proposed. Both the complexity and the rapid course of human growth suggest that multiple sources of influence are necessary for development to occur. Rather, this chapter emphasizes the important contribution that one source of influence—social experience—has in promoting cognitive growth.

WHAT ARE THE MECHANISMS OF COGNITIVE DEVELOPMENT?

All aspects of human development involve change. Emotional life changes and becomes more complex with age. Children are increasingly capable of producing, interpreting, and regulating a wider array of emotional experiences. Children's social life also transforms. The nature and number of children's relationships change, as does their skill at interacting with others. Intellectually, children increase their competence across a wide range of domains, including concept formation, reasoning, problem solving, remembering, and using language. What produces these changes and how does developmental theory account for them?

Developmental study makes a unique contribution to the field of psychology through its concentration on the processes and outcomes of change. Thus, for a theory to be a *developmental* theory, it must focus on changes in human behavior or thinking that occur over time. It must also include an explanation of how these changes occur (Miller, 1993). According to Flavell (1984), human development has two parts, or halves, what he calls the "how" and the "what" of development. For Flavell, the "how" may be the more important half for developmental psychologists to describe. This is because the "what" of development, that is, the content of the knowledge that children develop, varies tremendously across cultural contexts and historical eras of development.

In contrast, the "how" of development, that is, the ways in which developmental change occurs, may be invariant across individuals, contexts, and time periods, and thereby reflect a species-general property.

The term *mechanism* is used to describe the change process or processes underlying developmental achievements. A mechanism includes a set of general principles, or rules, that describe a developmental change. These principles include the *antecedents required for the change*, that is, what the organism must have in order for a particular development to occur. For instance, certain physical capabilities, like bone development, muscle strength, and balance, are needed before a child takes her first step. These, then, would be antecedents of this developmental change.

The set of principles describing change must also include the *motivating force or forces that generate the change*. These may be internal to the organism, as proposed in Freudian theory; external to the organism, as depicted in social learning theory; or result from some interaction between internal and external forces, as discussed by Piaget. The principles must also specify *factors that may influence or modify the change* in individual cases. Factors that affect change in an individual can be internal in origin, such as a genetic aberration, or external, such as educational opportunities.

Finally, principles of change must explain *why certain courses of development occur and others do not*. For example, Piaget explained why the development of logical reasoning would unfold in interaction with the physical world. He also explained why illogical reasoning would not develop. This is because illogic would lead to an unsatisfying cognitive consequence, a state he called "disequilibrium." For Piaget, humans are motivated to attain equilibrium between their understanding of the world and the logic that the world itself contains.

These criteria require much research to be satisfied. Thus most theoretical accounts of development fall short in some aspects. Whereas Piagetian theory provides a comprehensive description of some aspects of thinking that change with development, it does not explain in precise ways how these changes occur (Klahr, 1982). Information-processing and contextual approaches concentrate more on the mechanisms of change than they do on the content of development. Yet, even in these approaches, mechanisms are delineated better in some theories than in others. Specifying these gaps may help direct research in ways that enhance theoretical formulations. In addition, accurate accounts of mechanisms of change may enhance understanding of cognitive development in other ways.

Without an understanding of how change occurs, it is unclear what processes instigate and organize human intellectual development.

It is evident from observations, across the wide range of contexts in which people develop and in the many domains of functioning in which the mind is capable of performing competently, that cognitive development proceeds in an organized fashion. This suggests that a set of common principles underlies much of what occurs over the course of intellectual growth. However, because different contextual constraints lead to different overt behaviors, clearly described and specified mechanisms of change make it possible to examine whether changes that occur across different contexts, and appear different on the surface, actually stem from the same psychological process. Along these same lines, better understanding of mechanisms of change may help psychologists predict behavior outside the context in which an observation occurred. In other words, better understanding of developmental mechanisms not only enriches theory, it may also be useful for explaining when, where, and why certain behaviors appear or do not appear, and whether seemingly different behaviors share similar psychological underpinnings.

Despite great interest in the mechanisms of development, current understanding of change in all areas of developmental study is limited (Brown & DeLoache, 1978; Flavell, 1984; Miller, 1993; Siegler, 1996). In part this is due to the fact that mechanisms of change are not easy to observe. In addition, as Siegler (1996) has argued, understanding change may also be hampered by the tendency of researchers to characterize thinking and its development along simple dramatic lines that describe what children's thinking is like at different ages, the "what" of development, rather than what produces the changes that are observed. And, finally, when change is the focus of research, accounts of the mechanisms of change are often sketchy.

To counter these limitations, Miller (1993) suggests that future theories of development examine the two roles that developmental mechanisms play. First, theories should specify how a mechanism facilitates the acquisition of new skills. This has been the main emphasis in characterizing mechanisms of cognitive development in several theories, and includes notions like equilibration, learning, and strategy acquisition. Second, a complete explanation of mechanisms should include how cognitive skills are accessed (i.e., made available for use) in specific contexts. Questions about how children learn to apply the skills they have developed, and how skills that have been learned in one context are transferred or generalized to another context, are what is at issue here. According to Miller (1993), any particular mechanism of development may play one or both of these roles.

I hold the view that social experience can serve as a mechanism for cognitive development on both these counts. I describe research and theory that demonstrates how social partners help children develop new cognitive skills as well as deploy previously learned skills in new contexts. The social context affords children structured opportunities to practice, refine, and extend their thinking skills. Information provided by the social context, such as the assistance of other people and the material and symbolic tools available, help children transfer knowledge and skills that they have learned and practiced in one context to other problem situations. Thus, through social interaction and by involvement with the tools and resources of the social and cultural community, children develop cognitive skills. These experiences improve children's ability to process information and thereby interact with the world more effectively—a criterion that Siegler (1989) considers essential for a process to qualify as a mechanism of cognitive development.

A twofold purpose underlies this discussion of social experience as a mechanism of cognitive development. The first is to add social experience to the list of other mechanisms of cognitive change that have been previously identified (Siegler, 1989; Sternberg, 1984). The second is to examine research findings in a way that demonstrates how the social mechanism of cognitive change operates. To do this, I discuss research that points to developmental change in particular domains of cognitive development and that stems from social experience. This is intended to address a shortcoming in cognitive developmental research based on a social contextual approach. This research has tended to focus on the social processes involved rather than on the content of the change observed. However, both emphases are necessary in order for this approach to contribute to the field more broadly.

As forewarning, I must stress that this goal—that is, the goal of specifying the social mechanism of cognitive change across a range of domains of functioning—will not be satisfied completely. In many domains, there is little pertinent research. In other domains, the research that exists to support this claim was not conducted with this purpose in mind. Thus, one of my desired outcomes in this book is the identification of empirical investigations that are needed in order to specify further the principles that define a social mechanism of cognitive development.

This task is challenging. As Klahr (1982) has pointed out, it is one thing to identify a mechanism of change and quite another to describe in detail how it operates. In the course of this examination, Sternberg's (1984) cautionary note about describing mechanisms of cognitive change will serve as a guide. According to Sternberg (1984), many of the mechanisms that developmental theories rely on are essentially elaborate descriptions of an observation. These may include process terms—for example, integrating new information with previous knowledge, symbolically representing a concept, or detecting affordances. Yet these are not, in and of themselves, explanations of development. They are, for Sternberg, pseudomechanisms. Though they may suggest an explanation, more detail as to how they operate to create and direct change is needed. Sternberg argues that in order to qualify as a mechanism of developmental change, a process must go beyond an observation by being *generative,* that is, it must explain phenomena beyond that which the observation conveys. It must also be *bounded*: since no mechanism can explain all processes of development, the limits or boundaries of what can be explained must be defined.

Before I examine social experience as a mechanism of cognitive change, I will discuss other external factors that have been considered instrumental to cognitive development. The purpose of this discussion is to make clear the unique contribution to the field that consideration of social experience as a mechanism of cognitive change can offer.

WHAT EXTERNAL FACTORS HAVE BEEN IMPLICATED AS MECHANISMS OF COGNITIVE CHANGE?

Other than maturational views of intellectual development that rely exclusively on biological explanations of cognitive change, all theories of cognitive development assume that external or exogenous forces influence change in some way. This section concentrates on two main approaches to intellectual development, the Piagetian and the information-processing views. Although the field of cognitive development is far broader and more eclectic theoretically than this coverage represents, these two general approaches still organize the field to a large degree in relation to the mechanisms that are assumed to underlie development. Examination of these two approaches is therefore useful for orienting the reader to the types of external mechanisms of change that currently exist in the field.

Although Piagetian and information-processing approaches differ on many counts, some of which are covered below, one similarity exists. Neither view accounts in its theoretical structure for the role that the social world plays in cognitive development. Although it may be true that each of these views, in its own way, could incorporate a social mechanism of change in its theory, this has yet to be done. Typically, when research based on either of these perspectives incorporates social factors, findings are rarely used to reformulate the theory. Rather, they appear as exceptions or peculiarities waiting for later theoretical integration.

Piagetian Theory and External Mechanisms of Cognitive Change

Piaget argued that thinking develops in response to pressing internal demands to make sense of the world around us. In this view, the environment is informative, but exactly how it informs the child is dependent upon what the child currently knows and how he or she is capable of interacting with and constructing meaning from this experience.

To explain how this type of interaction functions as a vehicle for change, Piaget proposed the twin mechanisms of *assimilation* and *accommodation*. These two processes help the organism achieve equilibrium between what is known and what exists in the world. In assimilation, external data are fit with currently known ways of understanding, or *schemas*. In accommodation, schemas are altered to fit with external data. For Piaget, these dialectical processes are always present whenever learning occurs. Knowledge is constructed as individuals rely on these processes to fine-tune their current understanding in relation to incoming information from the world. The accumulation of constructed knowledge results in a "critical mass" of information which can then lead to development, assuming that biological readiness is also in place.

What types of external, or exogenous, influences are the focus of this approach? For Piagetian and some neo-Piagetian psychologists, equilibrium is achieved through the interaction of the organism and the physical properties and objects of the world. Essentially, this view posits a passive environment in which the organism actively constructs meaning. Piaget acknowledged the contribution of social experience to cognitive development in one regard. According to Piaget, conflict between partners may affect cognitive development. Recall that for Piaget the key impetus of cognitive growth is *disequilibrium,* that is, discordance between what the child knows and the information presented by the environment. Although Piaget stressed that disequilibrium is largely an intrapsychological process, he did contend that certain social arrangements could thrust a child into disequilibrium and thereby instigate mental growth as the child strives to reestablish equilibrium. Thus, a social agent may mediate the equilibrium–disequilibrium process by making evident to a child the mismatch between what is known and some state of the world. For Piaget, this occurs when peers close to but not identical in their understanding engage in cognitive conflict.

The process of cognitive conflict requires open communication in that one person needs to be free or confident enough in speaking to another person in a conflictual way, that is, a way that contradicts or criticizes the partner's current knowledge state. For this reason, Piaget considered social interaction between peers of almost equal status, "near-peers," as the ideal arrangement for such opportunities to emerge. The notion of "almost equal status" for Piaget pertains to the partner's knowledge state or status and not to other connotations of the term *status,* for example, socioeconomic status or popularity. For Piaget, there needs to be some disequilibrium in knowledge states in order for one partner to possess a more mature understanding than the other partner. This knowledge difference can then be used to lead the less knowledgeable partner toward a more mature, or equilibrated, way of understanding.

Other than cognitive conflict involving peers, most of Piaget's writings about developmental change concentrate on the interaction of the child with the physical properties and objects of the world. The reasons why Piaget focused on the physical properties of the environment are complex. In part they stem from his philosophical interests. He was especially influenced by the writings of Immanuel Kant (1724–1804) on the construction of a scientific theory of knowledge. Like Kant, Piaget was interested in logical, mathematical, and physical concepts. However, Piaget differed from philosophers interested in these topics in that he emphasized the role played by overt activities in building up, or constructing, the conceptual basis of thought. In other words, his focus was on the *ontological,* or developmental, processes that underlie human logic. To study these processes he investigated the child's and the adolescent's interaction with the physical and objective qualities of the environment.

Interestingly, some have argued that Piaget's lack of attention to social processes may even have affected his studies of physical concepts (Donaldson, 1978; Samuel & Bryant, 1984; Siegel, 1991). (Chapter 6 begins with an example from Piaget's research along these very lines.) The form of inquiry and the task materials he used in these studies have social properties, properties that he did not examine, but that nevertheless affected children's performance. In essence, social experience affects the ways in which children interact with, learn from, and demonstrate understanding of physical features of the environment.

Although developmental psychology has benefited tremendously from Piaget's investigations of these topics, it is also true that Piaget was insufficiently attentive to the social contributions to cognitive development. This omission led to formidable difficulties in his theory, especially in explaining the variability in formal operational reasoning across cultural communities and within Western societies (Rogoff, Gauvain, & Ellis, 1984). This view is also problematic in the examination of children's everyday reasoning in contrast to their performance on more constrained or controlled laboratory tasks. Since the settings in which children develop and use cognitive skills are "rich" in a social sense, in terms of both other people and of human-made resources, understanding cognitive development in the everyday world in which development occurs requires going beyond much of what is defined theoretically in Piagetian psychology.

As a final point, one more specific to the discussion of mechanisms, Piaget did not elaborate on the ways in which external influences organize and direct cognitive change. His processes of assimilation and accommodation are underspecified (Klahr, 1982), that is, he provided few details as to what they are and how they work. Thus, as models for ways of thinking about the relation of social experience and cognitive change, the mechanisms proposed by Piaget fall short. Proposals by neo-Piagetians, such as M-space (Pascual-Leone, 1970) and representational redescription (Karmiloff-Smith, 1995), are more detailed in this regard, but they still do not address in any central way the contribution of social experience to cognitive change. However, it is important to note that some researchers working from a neo-Piagetian perspective recognize the role that social interaction and other culturally mediated processes play in the development of thinking. For instance, Karmiloff-Smith (1995) writes that among the many influences on development, the child's sociocultural environment, experienced primarily through cultural tools and social interaction, is extremely important and maps on readily to the inherent flexibility and adaptive qualities of the human mental system.

Information-Processing Approaches and External Mechanisms of Cognitive Change

The second dominant approach to cognitive development is based on information-processing views of cognition. A number of developmental theories have been derived from this general approach. These theories are similar in that they all consider thinking as information processing, chiefly involving the acts of representing and operating on knowledge. However, because they are *developmental* theories, they emphasize how children represent and transform information over the course of growth. Of particular interest is how children of different ages operate on information to reach a goal and their capacity for organizing and storing this information.

A hallmark of information-processing approaches is their attention to change mechanisms. The two general sources of cognitive change that have been the focus of research are the acquisition of particular skills and increases in the capacity and rate of processing information (Miller, 1993). Several more specific mechanisms have been proposed, including automization (Case, 1992), regularity detection (Klahr, 1992), generalization (Klahr & Wallace, 1976), enhanced neural connections (MacWhinney, 1987), strategy construction (Sternberg, 1985), and strategy choice (Siegler, 1996). These processes contribute to change by modifying the cognitive system in ways that lead to differences in functioning, in most cases through more effective or more efficient ways of processing information.

Investigators of these processes have been attentive to external sources of influences on their development. Careful task analysis in laboratory situations, along with the use of models to simulate and predict processes of reasoning and how they change, are central to this overall approach. Little attention in this approach has been paid to the everyday context of development and how the mechanisms proposed operate in more natural settings (Neisser, 1982). In addition, as in Piagetian-based views, concern with external contributions to change has mainly focused on children's experience with the physical world. In some cases, the child's interaction with the world of symbols is the focus. But, as in the Piagetian work, such symbols are rarely connected to the social context from which they come and which gives them meaning.

In other words, despite extensive study of how a particular task may influence performance and learning, children's thinking in a task context is typically local in emphasis. By this I mean that the larger social and cultural context that provides meaning and purpose for the activity is virtually ignored. Recent forays into the ways in which information processing develops in more everyday contexts and practices may remedy this flaw, however (see, e.g., Sternberg & Wagner, 1986). Examination of thinking in its everyday context requires consideration of the broader social and cultural context of meaning in order to understand a task and a performance.

Also of interest to a sociocultural approach is the recent emphasis by Siegler (1996) on the role of variability and choice in developmental change. In his study of the different change mechanisms proposed across many theories of intellectual development, Siegler identified a core similarity in what on the surface appears to be a variety of disparate views: all include some way for organisms to produce variation in their behavior, variations that lead to specialized ways of thinking or acting in particular circumstances that, ideally, are adaptive for the organism. This observation led Siegler to suggest that *variability*—the potential to behave in one of a number of ways—and *choice*—the ability to choose intelligently among the alternatives available—are important to cognitive change. In other words, for Siegler, variability and choice facilitate the production of behaviors that support human adaptation. Because these behaviors are adaptive, they become built into (and thus change) the individual's behavioral repertoire. Development would, therefore, depend on the ability of the organism to select, and select reasonably well, among the various behavioral alternatives available in any given situation. This selection process involves coordinating what is already known about the circumstance with knowledge about what behaviors are available or potentially available and suited to the situation.

From a social contextual perspective, other people play fundamental roles in supporting children in this selection process. Children, whom Brown and De Loache (1978) call "universal novices," are frequently inexperienced and do not understand the range of behavioral choices available in a particular context. They also lack knowledge about which behaviors are more valued, important, or critical in the situation. Thus, behavioral choice poses serious challenges for children. These challenges are related to a child's developmental status, that is, the child's age. When children are very young, both their knowledge of the choices available and their ability to obtain a particular choice are restricted. Therefore, they can often only access a choice through the assistance of another person. As a case in point, developmentalists who study early social and emotional development are interested in how infants use the skills they have available to them, such as early smiling or vocalizing or orienting behaviors, to entice more mature partners into helping them attain a reasonable or acceptable course of action. Social–cognitive processes of intersubjectivity, joint attention, and social referencing (discussed in Chapter 4) are pivotal in these situations. Although toddlers have more access than infants to the choices available in a situation, they often do not know enough about the different alternatives—for example, what things they should avoid (hot or sharp items) or treat in special ways (delicate items)—and assistance from others is critical. Essentially, for young children, their mobility surpasses their ability to select well from the myriad of behavioral choices available in any particular context. As a result, other, more experienced individuals aid them in making these choices. As children get older, their skill across the many domains of cognitive functioning increases, as does their social contact with peers and adults outside the family system. However, their knowledge and access to resources is restricted in ways unique to their age group. Thus, across development, collaboration with peers and adults may take on different forms, but it continues to aid children in the selection and enactment of choices for action. Even during adolescence, when new relations with peers emerge, these social partners, with their own emerging social, cognitive, and emotional skills, play important roles in mediating the pattern of the adolescent's strategic behavior.

Thus, at each point in development, the question arises: How are age-related development and constraints in information processing co-ordinated with the assistance and support of the social world in ways that inform the child in choosing a particular course of action from the whole range of actions possible in a situation? From a sociocultural perspective, the social world helps bridge these "developmental" gaps, and is therefore a constituent mechanism in processing information. Together, the protracted path of human maturation and the unique sociohistorical circumstances of growth ensure that the social community is a vibrant part of how and what information is processed. This is the focus of the next section.

SOCIAL PROCESSES AS MECHANISMS OF INTELLECTUAL GROWTH

All human beings participate in organized patterns of social behavior. These patterns, and the transactions they afford, affect the opportunities that children have to develop and practice cognitive skills. Several social processes exert influence and direction on cognitive development. These include interpersonally direct processes like interaction in the child's zone of proximal development (Vygotsky, 1978) and guided participation (Rogoff, 1990). In addition, less interpersonally direct, yet still fundamentally social, processes also contribute to the development of cognitive skill. These processes include legitimate peripheral participation (Lave & Wenger, 1991) and the arrangement for and regulation of children's everyday activities (Gauvain, 1999). These social processes communicate to children the ways of thinking and behaving that are valued in their community and provide opportunities and support for developing these skills. A brief discussion of the child's active role in this process is useful for distinguishing this approach from social learning theory in which the child plays primarily a passive or reactive role.

The Active Role of the Learner in Social-Cognitive Transactions

Human beings create and participate in many social activities throughout the day that affect the course of intellectual development. For children, the majority of these activities are structured by more experienced members of the community in which the children develop. These people help children engage, from early in life, in the activities and routines of their social and cultural community. Both the adult and the child play active roles in this process. Furthermore, the process of development itself plays an active role. For learning to occur, these activities must be coordinated with the emerging skills and capabilities of the child.

Consider the game of peekaboo, a form of play found in many communities throughout the world. This game draws on the infant's emerging skills of responsiveness, anticipation, and object knowledge. The adult coordinates the infant's skills with the rule structure of the game in a process called *social synchronization* (Bruner & Sherwood, 1976). This process, facilitated by the strong emotional and social bonds between the parent and the infant, changes as the child develops. An important developmental achievement from experience with the game of peekaboo is that the child learns the basic rules of the game, as well as variations of these rules. For example, the act of uncovering the face is the main feature of the game. This activity is open to substantial variation: sometimes the unmasking is controlled by the mother, sometimes by the child, and sometimes the mother prompts the child to uncover whatever is masking her face. Bruner and Sherwood observed that when an infant is younger than 12 months of age, most of the unmasking is controlled by the mother. After the child is 12 months of age, he or she assumes more responsibility for this act.

For Bruner and Sherwood (1976), this type of ritualized play is a stepping-stone in cognitive development. Infants learn the rules of play. They also learn that variation, even within a constrained set of rules, is possible, even desirable. This understanding is critical to the child's developing competence in this and other contexts. But in order for this process to work, the active engagement of both participants is essential. For the child, active participation includes his or her motivation, enjoyment, and interest in the activity, as well as feedback to the partner about what the child already knows and whether the new information is understood and of continued interest.

Children's active role in procuring and maintaining information derived from social experience appears very early in life. Research by Collie and Hayne (1999) shows that children as young as 6 months of age can learn new behaviors simply by observing the actions of others, even for as little as 30 seconds. Researchers used hand puppets and other attractive toys to engage the infants' attention, and then assessed how long infants were able to remember what they had seen as well as their ability to imitate these actions on their own. At 6 months of age, infants were able to retain these memories for a day; at 12 months, they retained the information for a week; at 18 months they retained it for as long as a month.

Over the course of development, children's active engagement in social–cognitive processes reflects their changing competence as well as the type of cognitive skills that are of interest or challenging to them as particular points of growth. In the preschool years, one of the noticeable changes that occurs in children's thinking is their ability to understand and use symbols—for example, symbolic representations like step-by-step plans for making objects (Gauvain, de la Ossa, & Hurtado, 1996). Learning how to understand and use plans is a rather complex task for children. More experienced partners are needed to provide support for this learning. The following exchange between a mother and her 4-year-old child while they used a plan to construct a toy illustrates the active role of the child in this type of learning.

MOTHER: Now you need another one like this on the other side. Mmmmmm . . . there you go, just like that.

SADIE: Then I need this one to go like this? Hold on, hold on. Let it go. There. Get that out. Oops!

MOTHER: I'll hold it while you turn it. (*Watches Sadie work on toy.*) Now you make the end.

SADIE: This one?

MOTHER: No, look at the picture. Right here (*points to plan*). That piece.

SADIE: Like this?

MOTHER: Yeah.

Here the child is learning to use a plan to guide action and her mother is assisting her in this process. The mother regulates the difficulty of the child's involvement and the child informs the mother as to whether the task is manageable and understood.

During middle childhood children are developing metacognitive skills and strategies for solving problems. Social–cognitive experiences are important here as well. Consider Ben's description, at 6½ years of age, to his mother of his efforts to teach chess, a game that Ben's father had been teaching him, to his friend Robert.

BEN: I tried to play as hard as I could because this helps the learner learn faster because he'll say "Hey, that's not fair" and try harder. I just learned that today. I wonder if Dad knows that.

MOTHER: What?

BEN: When Daddy taught me how to play checkers he always played soft on me. When he played soft I always won. But if he didn't play soft, he would win. If the learner doesn't know how to play very good, you play as hard as you can and it makes them concentrate and look at the board.

These comments suggest that Ben learned something about strategies from playing these games with others. He also derived some understanding of how to teach these games to others. Whether or not he was effective when he instructed the other child is not known. But what is clear is that he drew conclusions about teaching and learning from a social experience and that this information was not explicitly taught to him. In other words, when his father taught him how to play checkers, he learned the rules of the game. But he also learned something else: he learned about teaching the game. Furthermore, he was able to generalize this knowledge from one game (checkers) to another game (chess). In essence, he was able to derive a more general principle about learning and games from this social experience, namely, that playing in a challenging or "hard" way with a new player may lead to more effective learning. It is also interesting that this observation or insight led him to wonder if his father knew this principle, since, in Ben's estimation, his father's behavior suggested that he did not. Ben not only displayed some awareness of his own thinking processes, he demonstrated cognizance that others also have thinking processes.

These examples illustrate the active role of the child at different points in development in social–cognitive transactions. They also illustrate that what children can learn from social interaction is cognitive in nature, such as learning how to use a symbolic tool or to play a game or to deploy a strategy. It is important to stress that this type of knowledge can only be obtained through social interaction and is not available to children when they work on their own. Rules of play are *social* conventions; symbolic representations are *social* constructions; and modes of interaction, such as instruction, are *social* processes. Finally, these examples suggest that opportunities for cognitive development can and do emerge spontaneously and frequently in adult–child, especially parent–child, interaction. This does not imply, however, that these experiences always occur or lead to positive outcomes. For instance, the variations of a game presented to an infant can, in some cases, be overwhelming. In one mother–child pair observed by Bruner and Sherwood (1976), the mother introduced a large number of variations of the peekaboo game to the child. She also, at times, misread the child's cues. Over the course of the study, this dyad was unable to develop workable rules of play. Sometimes the mother would begin the game too soon, before the child was paying attention. Sometimes the person responsible for unmasking the mother was not clear or disputed. Research on parent–child interaction using plans also contained variation across dyads that was directly tied to the type of engagement by one or both participants (Gauvain et al., 1996). Whereas some dyads worked together smoothly and children's learning was evident, some dyads had a more bumpy course as mothers conveyed confusing messages about the plan or the child refused to use the plan to make the toy. Observations of dyadic exchanges between children and mothers with depressive symptoms (Goldsmith & Rogoff, 1995) and between mothers and chronically noncompliant preschoolers (Gauvain & De-Ment, 1991) also indicate that in certain dyads social–cognitive transactions do not necessarily proceed in positive directions. Although research has emphasized the beneficial role that social interaction may play in cognitive development, I must point out that such opportunities may be more frequent in some dyads than in others. This is because the active contributions of the participants influence the opportunities for children to learn in social contexts. The next section explores learning in social context further by examining several social processes that can support and lead cognitive development.

SOCIAL PROCESSES OF COGNITIVE DEVELOPMENT

Older and more experienced members of society help shape intellectual growth through the interactions they have with younger, less experienced members. These interactions influence intellectual development in terms both of how children think and of what they learn to think about. Through social interaction, more experienced members pass onto less experienced members the practices, values, and goals of the community. This process, which can be called *cognitive socialization,* relies on the inherent linkage between the larger sociocultural context of development and the more immediate or local circumstances of individual growth. In other words, the sociocultural context of development is instantiated in local social situations in the ways in which people interact and the areas of mental functioning that are stressed and rewarded. In this way, social interaction helps organize the developing mind in ways that are suited to the needs and aspirations of the community in which growth occurs. Social contact with more experienced cultural members allows for the transmission of culturally valued skills through collaboration in the child's zone of proximal development (Vygotsky, 1978), through the process of guided participation (Rogoff, 1990), and via less direct but still fundamentally social processes like legitimate peripheral participation (Lave & Wenger, 1991) and the provision and regulation of children's everyday activities (Gauvain, 1999).

Collaboration in the Zone of Proximal Development

Vygotsky (1978) considered the capability to engage in higher psychological functions the distinguishing feature of human psychology. To investigate this issue he adopted a developmental approach, insisting that psychological phenomena be studied as processes in motion and change. According to Vygotsky, higher mental functions can only be understood as dynamic processes that embody their own individual and social history as well as their own potential. For Vygotsky, "to study something historically means to study it in the process of change . . . [in order] to discover its nature, its essence, for it is only in movement that a body shows what it is" (p. 65).

According to Vygotsky (1978), higher mental functions have their origin in human social life as children interact with more experienced members of their community. This process involves a child as an active participant working with a more competent partner to solve a problem. To facilitate children's participation and learning, more experienced partners target their assistance to a child's *zone of proximal or potential development*, which is defined as "the distance between the actual developmental level as determined by independent problem solving and the level of potential development as determined through problem solving under adult guidance or in collaboration with more capable peers" (Vygotsky, 1987, p. 86). The key issue here is that the child's prospective accomplishments can be used as an index of development. That is, what the child is capable of knowing, thinking, or doing with appropriate support is, for Vygotsky, what cognitive development is all about. This is quite different from approaches that emphasize what the child is already capable of doing on his or her own, which Vygotsky considered as already developed (he referred to these as "fossilized behaviors"), and therefore as not particularly useful for describing the future course of development.

Interaction in the child's zone of proximal development involves exposing children to increasingly more complex understanding and activity than they are capable of on their own. Thus, the more experienced partner encourages and supports a child in using his or her current capabilities to extend the child's skill to higher levels of competence. New ways of thinking are first experienced collaboratively; only after this collaborative experience are they experienced individually. In other words, understanding occurs initially on the social plane and then later, after the child internalizes this understanding, on the individual plane. Thus, for Vygotsky, learning precedes development as the interpsychological becomes the intrapsychological.

Vygotsky's (1978) claim that higher mental functions originate in human social life is a strong one. Structural and organizational properties of human social interaction are considered reflections of the larger social context in which they are embedded. These properties shape the process of communication that occurs between people, and this, in turn, directly influences the individual psychological functioning that emerges from these social exchanges. This view implies that variation in interpsychological functioning should lead to differences in individual psychological functioning. Much of the research included later in this book on the zone of proximal development is directed toward this question.

The structure provided in communication serves as a "scaffold" (Wood & Middleton, 1975) for the learner, providing contact between old and new knowledge. In this way, the social world provides the child with *cognitive opportunities*—opportunities that originate in and are maintained through the contributions and goals of the participants— that encourage and support learning and growth. The process of jointly constructing and sharing meaning among individuals is called *intersubjectivity* (Rommetveit, 1974). Intersubjectivity involves cognitive, social, and emotional interchange, and makes possible the type of interaction that fosters the development of cognitive skill in social context. More experienced partners rely on a variety of social interactional techniques to support and encourage children's involvement in the zone. These techniques include suggestions, prompts, hints, directives, questions, praise, and demonstration. Researchers have assessed how these communication devices influence children's emerging understanding, as well as how adults' use of these tools changes over the course of an interaction. As this suggests, language and its development play central roles in all social approaches to cognitive development (Nelson, 1996). Language transforms how a person understands and acts upon the world. It enables the thinker to operate independently of immediate perceptual experiences and contemplate what cannot be seen, as well as to consider the past and the future.

Through the use of language and the presentation and arrangement of a joint activity, cognitive opportunities that arise as children and more experienced partners collaborate in the child's zone of proximal development benefit cognitive growth. This occurs because the learning situation can be uniquely tailored to the needs and skills of the learner as revealed over the course of the interaction. Growth is evident in the child's changing participation. Over time, as understanding is passed on from the teacher to the learner, the learner assumes more responsibility for solving the problem at hand (Rogoff, 1998).

The notion of the zone of proximal development has inspired research on the transmission of cognitive skill during social interaction involving an adult and child or peers. Results generally support the assertion that social experience can facilitate cognitive development (Rogoff, 1990). The notion of the zone of proximal development has also been used to study the organization of instruction in more formal learning situations. In their research on reading comprehension,

Palinscar and Brown (1984) demonstrated that when a tutor adjusts instruction to a child's current level of understanding, the child's comprehension skills are enhanced. This research led to the development of a tutorial method called *reciprocal teaching* that has had substantial impact on the educational community.

Vygotsky's idea of the zone of proximal development concentrates primarily on cognitive change and the mechanisms that underlie it. It postulates a social mechanism of change in that experience with other people is hypothesized as leading to a reorganization or restructuring of a child's current understanding. As children engage in increasingly more complex activities in social context, their understanding and participation changes, and a transformation in their cognitive approach to the problem or type of problem results. This conception of cognitive change is *microgenetic* in scope: it concentrates on change over a short period of time that is task-specific. That is, similar to much research based on an information-processing approach, change is defined in relation to a particular task, problem, or activity. Developmental change that reflects more *ontogenetic*, or age-related, growth is not directly implicated in the notion of the zone of proximal development, nor are results assumed to generalize across domains of understanding or of skill. As in information-processing approaches, these are considered shortcomings of Vygotsky's view (Miller, 1993). Finally, Vygotsky's description of functioning in the zone of proximal development largely concentrates on how the more experienced partner provides a child with a supportive context for learning. Vygotsky was less attentive to the learner's involvement and how this participation can be understood in cognitive developmental terms. However, as discussed above, active participation by learners is directly related to the cognitive opportunities and development that may result from social interaction. For example, descriptions of the process of scaffolding, in which adults support children's intellectual activity during social interaction, have tended to focus on the adult's contribution to this process and consequently to reduce the child to little more than the recipient of the adult's efforts. In her writings on guided participation, Rogoff (1990, 1996, 1998) provides a fuller account of the learner in the social–cognitive process.

Guided Participation

In order to account for the child's active role in procuring or appropriating understanding through social interaction, as well as to emphasize other social arrangements that contribute to cognitive development, Rogoff (1990) introduced the notion of *guided participation*. In this view, cognitive change results as children participate in intelligent ac-

tion alongside more experienced partners. Over the course of participation, as a child's roles and responsibilities in joint action change, the
child's understanding of the task also changes (Rogoff, 1996). In this
view, the child is not merely a learner, that is, a naive actor who follows
the instructions or prompts of the more experienced partner. Rather,
the child is a full participant, albeit a participant of a specific type characterized by individual and developmentally related skills, interests, resources, and so forth. The development of children's thinking through
guided participation reflects the child's developmental status as the
child's current and emerging understanding and skills determine the
roles and responsibilities the child assumes.

In this view, children's participation in the organized routines and
practices of the social community contribute right alongside more didactic interactional experiences to cognitive development. To support
her view, Rogoff discusses cross-cultural evidence that indicates developmental change that coincides with children's changing involvement
in the community (see, e.g., Weisner, 1996; Whiting & Edwards, 1988).
One interesting source of evidence along these lines follows the conceptualization put forward by Mead (1935, 1949) in her age-related
classification of children as lap children, knee children, yard children,
and community or school-age children. These descriptors characterize
development as a process of changing participation both in the settings
children occupy and the social relations they form. Research by Mead
and other anthropologists along these lines (see, e.g., Munroe &
Munroe, 1971; Whiting & Edwards, 1988) highlights the social consequences of these developmentally related experiences. Rogoff (1990)
draws attention to the cognitive consequences of these changes.

This approach to describing cognitive development is quite different from the more common approach in psychological research in
which the description of children's age-related performances on solitary laboratory tasks is paramount. For Rogoff, the process of guided
participation shifts the level of psychological analysis away from the individual child per se toward the child's changing participation in socially organized activity.

Indirect Social Experience and Cognitive Development

Every society organizes the environment and routines of children in order to shape development in ways that are beneficial for the community. Because all humans have similar basic needs, the routines of daily
life, especially for the young, have much commonality across cultural
communities. Despite commonalities, the ways in which routines are
carried out varies depending upon socialization goals. These variations
may influence the development of all types of cognitive skills.

One way in which social experiences other than direct social interaction and guided participation may affect cognitive development is
through opportunities for children to observe mature behaviors in
their community. Lave and Wenger (1991) emphasize the role of observation in exposing children, or less experienced cultural members, to
more experienced members as they participate in valued cultural practices (see also Goodnow, Miller, & Kessel, 1995). This process, which is
called *legitimate peripheral participation*, may be especially important in
settings in which explicit adult–child instruction is less common than in
Western communities.

For Lave and Wenger, the central point is that not all developmentally related skills are learned by direct guidance or by instruction.
Rather, much learning occurs as children live alongside others who are
participating in and thereby demonstrating culturally valued skills. This
process is similar to the type of social modeling described by Bandura
(1986), but it differs in that it emphasizes the cultural and goal-directed
nature of these transactions and the active role of the learner in the
process. An example of legitimate peripheral participation is provided
by Greenfield (1984) in her discussion of the transmission of weaving
skills from expert to novice weavers among the Zinacantecans, a Mayan
community in Mexico. Greenfield and Childs (1991) found that much
of this skill was transferred across generations as apprentice weavers
stood quietly alongside and watched more experienced individuals, like
their mothers and older sisters, weave.

Other less interpersonally direct but still fundamentally social processes also contribute to the acquisition and organization of individual
cognitive skills. Social processes, such as the determination of children's daily routines, play materials, activity settings, and companions,
compose a substantial portion of the cognitive opportunities that children encounter in their everyday lives (Gauvain, 1999). In fact, the primary power that parents and other more experienced community
members exert over cognitive development, especially in the years after
infancy, may not be in direct dyadic exchanges with children. Rather, it
may be through control over the network composition and boundaries
of children's social and mental lives (Parke & Bhavnagri, 1989; Whiting, 1980).

Consideration of less direct social processes as mechanisms of cognitive development puts the spotlight on children's everyday experiences as opportunities for cognitive development. It extends Rogoff's
view of guided participation by defining the socially organized nature
of children's everyday activities that, in addition to more direct dyadic
exchanges, may contribute to children's emerging skills at thinking and
problem solving. Variation exists in the ways in which children are involved in the mature practices of their community (Goodnow et al.,

1995; Morelli, Rogoff, & Angelillo, 1993; Whiting & Edwards, 1988), with patterns reflecting both short- and long-term goals and values of the community. These variations would be expected to lead to differences in what children learn to think about and how they learn to think.

These experiences may effect cognitive development in a number of ways. They provide children with an introduction to and practice in activities that foster the development of particular cognitive skills. They provide children with opportunities to observe more experienced participants as models for future action (legitimate peripheral participation). This may emerge in informal encounters as well as more formal arrangements, like apprenticeships. They provide children with experiences using tools and artifacts, both material and symbolic, that are derived from the sociocultural context of development. Each of these experiences relies on the active role of children and adults in culturally based practices that afford opportunity for the development of cognitive skill. In this way, the sociocultural context of development is seen as providing the core activities through which children are exposed to and learn about thinking.

CONCLUDING THOUGHTS

The two primary theoretical approaches to the study of cognitive development, Piagetian and information-processing views, do not attend to the single most ubiquitous and influential external resource available to the growing mind: other people. Additionally, findings based on interactions with the physical world cannot be readily extrapolated to social interactional processes. Social experiences are not resources for cognitive development in the same way as things in the physical world. Unlike the physical world, the social world provides the developing mind with a dynamic and mutually generated context that originates in and is maintained by the contributions and goals of the participants. Involvement with others, either at play or at work, creates opportunities for individuals to evaluate and refine their understanding as they are exposed to the thinking of others and as they participate in creating shared understanding. In this way, social experience can serve as a mechanism for developmental change.

For those who study the role of the social context in cognitive development, social processes not only affect children's experience in that setting, they also contribute in formative ways to the development and organization of thinking. In other words, experience with other people is considered instrumental in the formation and developmental course of human intelligence. For obvious reasons, these experiences are particularly influential in domains of functioning that rely on understanding that is primarily socially generated and shared. However, what is easily overlooked is the fact that this includes most of the higher level mental functions. These functions rely in fundamental ways on the integration of individual thinking with the symbolic or representational tools that have been devised and passed on by the social community. This integration forms the social foundation of cognitive development.

A social approach to cognitive development introduces a different level of analysis into research, namely, socially constituted cognitive activity. Socially constituted cognitive activity is individual thinking that has embedded within it the contributions of the social world. This approach proposes mechanisms of cognitive change that are overlooked in other theoretical accounts. The social processes discussed in this chapter are the object of much current research on cognitive development. Part II of this book concentrates on this research. Although these processes have been shown in many ways to provide opportunities for, and thereby to promote, cognitive development, it also appears that they may impose constraints on cognitive development. However, it is presently unclear how cognitive interaction constrains cognitive activity and what the consequences of these constraints may be for cognitive development. As Goodnow (1987) has noted, interaction in the zone is not always a benign process. In some cases it may open doors, as parents or teachers and learners grow together. In others, it may pose limits on what children learn or on how they learn. Better understanding of the ways in which social interaction provides opportunities and constraints for cognitive growth is needed. To do this requires attention to the socioemotional context of the interaction, along with the shared social history of a dyad (Gauvain & DeMent, 1991; Gauvain & Fagot, 1995), both of which are discussed at various points throughout this book. It is also important to stress that examination of the social contribution to cognitive development may advance understanding of other mechanisms of cognitive development that have been proposed, such as Siegler's (1996) concepts of variability and choice. Social contextual research on children's thinking may point to the essential role that social partners play in supporting these proposed mechanisms of change.

An important, and potentially quite valuable, consequence of better integration of a social approach in the study of cognitive development is that investigators cannot restrict themselves to the study of people growing up in one setting or even in one historical period. If one wants to understand individual human cognition, it becomes important to examine the social forces that influenced its development, as well as the history of the mediational means that play a role in defining the cognitive processes that are used or not used in any particular setting in which intelligent behavior is displayed. In order to explore this linkage further, the next chapter discusses the sociocultural context of cognitive development.

Chapter 3

The Sociocultural Context
of Cognitive Development

To describe the social context of cognitive development more fully, in this chapter I discuss the sociocultural context of development in a way that ties it directly to human thinking and cognitive development. The social context of development is sometimes described without attention to the cultural system of meaning that underlies social experience, but this method substantially limits our understanding of cognitive development. This is because human beings live and learn to think in environments transformed by the accomplishments, symbolic systems, and artifacts of prior generations extending back to the beginning of the species (Geertz, 1973; Sahlins, 1976). The basic function of these human creations is to help human beings to interact with the physical world and with each other. Cultural tools contribute to this interaction via the support they provide for thinking. In addition to creating and using tools or techniques to support thinking, such as a knot in a rope or another type of mnemonic device to aid remembering, human beings also make these resources available to other human beings, especially new members of the community. Hence, each generation inherits a culture that has been modified by the accumulated resources for thinking and acting that were successful for prior generations of the group (Cole, 1996). Much of social interaction, especially for young or inexperienced members of a community, involves their introduction to and refinement of these symbolic and material tools in order to support and enhance mental activities.

Although the primary focus of this book is on how social processes, in particular social interaction, contribute to cognitive change, an implicit assumption of this view is that these social processes reflect the values, goals, and practices of the cultural community within which they are embedded and which give them meaning. Therefore, central to my discussion of how social experience functions as a mechanism of cognitive change is the role that culture plays in organizing human social experience, especially the interactional and symbolic experiences that children and adults share every day.

In order to draw out this connection, I will describe a theoretical approach—*activity theory*—that takes as its main focus the sociocultural nature of intellectual development. Activity theory, devised by psychologists working in Russia in the early and midpart of the 20th century, concentrates on organized human activity, especially people's goals and the means they use to attain these goals, as the primary level of psychological analysis. Although most of the research I present in later chapters was not conducted from the vantage point of activity theory, I will use the main tenets of this view to identify organized features of the social context that may be instrumental to cognitive growth. Activity theory does not provide a complete description of this process, however. Therefore, I also include a discussion of the limitations of this view for explaining cognitive development in social context. This critique may help clarify what needs to be added to this activity-based approach in order to advance understanding of a social mechanism of cognitive change. Following this discussion, I turn to an examination of the social resources involved in cognitive development. Other people serve as agents of cognitive socialization. For young children, the primary agents are family members, especially parents and siblings. As children get older, peers assume a more important role.

COGNITIVE DEVELOPMENT IN CULTURAL CONTEXT

Two important questions can be asked about mental development. The first, the most familiar to researchers, is How does the mind as an organized system function and grow? The second question, tied to the first, asks How does the individual mind connect with the minds of others? Human beings are social animals and the connections between individuals are a critical aspect of mental life. These connections not only help organize and sustain the human intellect, they also serve as templates for cognitive growth.

Consider this simple observation. In *all* societies *everywhere* in the world, *most* children grow up to be competent members of their communities. This impressive phenomenon is dependent on many factors. The most central is an inherent human ability to develop intellectual and social skills adapted to the circumstances in which growth occurs. It also relies on social and cultural practices that support and maintain desired patterns of development. In other words, cognitive development is the process by which basic biological capabilities are shaped in ways that fit with the social context in which these capabilities will be used. In essence, the human biological system is coordinated with the social context in ways that ensure certain patterns of growth. This remarkable coordination is not coincidental. These constituent elements of human development "grew up" together over the course of human evolutionary history (Donald, 1991).

A sociocultural approach to cognitive development brings this connection more clearly into view by attending to the social forces that help shape human intelligence and the social and cultural conditions in which human intelligence operates. According to this approach to cognitive development, to understand intellectual development it is essential to investigate the role that social experience plays in this process, as well as how, over the course of development, the social world becomes a constituent element of individual functioning.

This perspective concentrates on development because it is in the process of growth, from conception through adulthood, that we witness a remarkable collaboration between the social world and the individual. Participation in the social world organizes and provides meaning for individual human action and development. Through a complex fit between individual capabilities and social practices, individuals come to function in the formal and informal institutions and relationships they encounter throughout their lives. In other words, the sociocultural context of development—that is, the values, goals, and practices of the community—is instantiated in local social situations via the ways in which people interact and the areas of mental functioning that are stressed and rewarded in these settings and transactions. These are geared toward the skills and knowledge that are considered mature and competent in that setting.

Becoming Competent: A Sociocognitive Process

How do children develop the skills and knowledge to become competent members of their community? Human beings learn to think about and solve problems in their everyday lives through the appropriation, use, and adaptation of social practices and material and symbolic tools developed by their culture (Cole, 1996; Rogoff, 1998; Vygotsky, 1978; Wertsch, 1985). These practices and tools are passed onto children through the many social experiences they have every day. Adults and other more experienced partners play key roles in defining and modeling these practices and tools for children. These social experiences contain the tacit, underlying goal of ensuring that children, who will become the next generation of the community, will develop the skills and understanding necessary for mature participation in the community. Children play an active, directive role in this process as their developing capabilities set the stage and establish the boundaries for development within social context (Rogoff, 1990; Whiting & Edwards, 1988). Through these transactions, children and adults co-construct understanding (Valsiner, 1989), and this in turn fosters the development of children's thinking along socially and culturally desired lines.

A focus on the social contributions to cognitive development does not imply that internal, biological contributions are unimportant. Although in this book I adopt the view that cognitive development is fundamentally a social process, I consider cognitive development to be a product of the coordination of human biology, both in terms of capabilities and constraints, and the values, opportunities, and goals of the social community. These two contributions to development, the biological and the social, inform and refine each other over time. Cole (1996) has referred to them wisely as our "dual legacy" as human beings.

It is important to note that the idea that biological and social processes jointly contribute to cognitive development is not unique to a sociocultural approach. It also appears in recent developmental theory that emphasizes the biological constraints underlying human cognitive development. For instance, Gelman and Greeno (1989) state that the sociocultural environment has developed over time in ways that take advantage of the biological constraints of the organism. Likewise, Karmiloff-Smith (1995) acknowledges the interaction of *endogenous,* or biological, factors, and *exogenous* factors, chiefly sociocultural interaction patterns, in the development of certain aspects of mental functioning. A sociocultural approach differs from these views in placing greater emphasis on the social and cultural processes that provide opportunities for cognitive development. Of particular concern is defining the linkage between individual cognitive performance and the social and cultural values and practices on which the performance relies.

In sum, the sociocultural view holds that the values, practices, and goals of a culture are revealed to children over time in the context of local situations. Proponents of this view recognize it would be a mistake to ignore the overarching developmental goals implicit in these activities. Local social experiences compose the individual units of the larger set of purposeful directed actions that carry people through the day. For children, these experiences are directed, more-or-less depending upon the event, to the goal of becoming a mature community member. Over the span of development children are expected to come to an understanding of and master the mature practices of their community. Some of these are unique to the historical and/or social circumstances of the community, while many others are similar to practices of neighboring communities or communities with similar socialization goals, and still more reflect biologically based requirements that are universal to the species. This stance suggests that questions about the origins and development of the mind in social context are as central to the study of cognitive development as are questions about the biological foundation of the mind. The biological underpinnings of the mind and the social context in which the mind expresses itself are, essentially, two sides of the same coin. As one cannot imagine the human social world existing as it does without the biological "hardware" that humans possess, one also cannot imagine human intelligence separately from the social context that provides it with direction and meaning.

IDENTIFYING THE ORIGINS OF HIGHER MENTAL FUNCTIONS IN SOCIAL ACTIVITY

In an attempt to lay out the foundation of a developmental and psychological approach that can account for social mechanisms of cognitive change, I turn now to the theoretical perspective of activity theory. Key ideas in this perspective appear promising for explicating the social foundation of cognitive development. Before describing activity theory, I must point out that this perspective is not a theory in the sense that it proposes specific and falsifiable predictions (Altman & Rogoff, 1987). It is more of a conceptual framework or a worldview about how to approach psychology and human development. It is expected that different theories may emerge from this view; indeed, some of the same assumptions are implicit in Bronfenbrenner's (1979) ecological approach, Gibson's (1979) perceptual theory, Lewin's (1964) field theory, Riegel's (1979) dialectical approach, and action theory (see, e.g., Frese & Sabini, 1985; Harre, 1984). I also need to stress that activity theory is not a monolithic view (Cole, 1996). There are theoretical disputes among those who study sociohistorical psychology and those who study the psychological theory of activity. The characterization of activity theory described below combines elements of these two related perspectives, and is consistent with the synthesis suggested by Zinchenko (1995). This synthesis describes social and cultural influences on cognitive development in a way that permits psychological examination across contexts. These ideas may, therefore, be useful for explicating both the opportunities and the constraints for cognitive growth that are inherent in the everyday activities in which children participate over the course of development.

Activity Theory

In the 1920s the Russian psychologist Lev S. Vygotsky (1962, 1978, 1987) created an approach to studying human development that emphasized the role of social and cultural experience in the formation of higher mental functions. This approach is known as activity theory. Since Vygotsky's early writings, it has been advanced by others, notably Leont'ev (1981), Luria (1976), and Zinchenko (1981). In recent years there has been increasing interest among psychologists outside of Russia in the ideas of Vygotsky and activity theory (Wertsch & Tulviste, 1994). A number of scholars, including Bruner (1985), Cole (1985), Rogoff and Wertsch (1984), and Wertsch (1981, 1985), have been involved in introducing these ideas to psychologists and educators in the United States and Western Europe.

According to Wertsch (1985), the notion of activity as an analytical device is useful for studying human consciousness in social and cultural contexts. Because activities and the settings in which they occur are created by the participants in that setting, they reflect the assumptions, the resources, and the goals of the group. This notion transcends the boundary between the individual and the social. In so doing, it connects the interpsychological plane, that is, *between* individuals, and the intrapsychological plane, that is, *within* an individual, of human functioning and development. Activity theory is based on three premises: (1) behavior is goal-directed and practical, (2) development is a product of social and cultural history, and (3) cognition is a socially mediated process.

Goal-Directed Nature of Human Behavior

Activity theory emphasizes the functional or practical nature of human action as people conduct purposeful goal-directed activities (Leont'ev, 1981; Vygotsky, 1978). The developmental implication is that children learn about and practice thinking in the course of participating in goal-directed activities—activities defined and organized by the cultural community in which development occurs. Much psychological research has focused on the organized, goal-directed nature of human activity, for example, Duncker's (1945) classic studies of functional fixedness and Bartlett's studies of memory (1932) and thinking (1958), so this basic idea is not new. What is new is (1) an emphasis on the connection between activity structure (the means and the goals that define human action) and the cultural practices from which they stem, and (2) an examination of the relations among activity structures, cultural practices, and cognitive growth. According to this view, neither mind nor behavior alone should be the primary unit of analysis in psychological study. Rather, the primary unit of study should be socially organized human activity (Leont'ev, 1981) in which individual psychological functions like perceiving, remembering, problem solving, conceptualizing, using language, and so forth work together to create meaningful action.

Research on children's everyday use of mathematics illustrates this linkage. Studies of the mathematical skills of Brazilian children who sell candy in the street (Carraher, Carraher, & Schliemann, 1985; Saxe, 1991) have found that these children can perform complex arithmetic operations that are related to the practice of selling candy, including adjustments for selling candy in unit amounts and for inflation. However, these same children are less skilled at these types of operations when they are presented in a more abstract or decontextualized form, which is how they appear in school. Findings such as these suggest that mental activity reflects the practices in which individuals engage, that these practices are defined by cultural convention and routine, and that such activities are handled differently and more successfully when the goal of the calculation is meaningful to the actor.

As another illustration, consider how cultural goals may organize social practices that may, in turn, affect cognitive activity. The values of cooperation and competition have been studied in Western and non-Western communities. In one study on this topic, Mackie (1983) compared European–New Zealand children and Maori children on a set of Piagetian tasks. These two groups differ in the extent to which they value cooperation in social activity, with the Maori placing greater value on cooperation. Even though Piaget hypothesized that conflict would lead to cognitive growth, a point that has been supported in research with Europeans and children of European ancestry, Mackie showed that Maori children were less likely to benefit from conflict.

Development as a Product of Social and Cultural History

Activity theory also stresses the idea that human psychological growth is a product of the cultural and social history in which an individual participates. Vygotsky was concerned with the influence of history on psychological development in several ways (Scribner, 1985). He was concerned with how general cultural history, that is, material resources and socially organized activities, promote human psychological functioning. He was also concerned with how a person's individual, or ontological, history, which contains both biological processes that regulate the development of basic mental functions and the sociocultural processes that regulate the development of higher mental functions, affect intellectual development. And, finally, he was interested in how the child's individual history and his or her social and cultural history merge to produce thinking. Thus, Vygotsky was concerned not only with transitions in individual development, that is, the individual's history, but also with changes that accrue over many individuals and generations and the convergence of the two.

Research on the use of particular cultural tools and the development of mathematical thinking illustrates this view. People who are skilled at using the abacus employ a "mental abacus" when calculating solutions in their heads (Hatano, Miyake, & Binks, 1977), and this skill enhances their mental calculation. Those skilled with pencil and paper calculations but not skilled with the abacus are less adept at mental calculation (Stigler, 1984; Stigler, Chalip, & Miller, 1986). How might this pattern have come about? Historical examination provides some insight into this psychological and developmental process (Swetz, 1987).

Late in the 12th century, a book by Leonardo of Pisa (also known as Fibonacci) introduced the West to Hindu–Arabic notation and described the commercial applications of this system. This idea was picked up by Italian merchants in the next century and led, in fairly short order, to changes in the conventions of calculating. In Europe at the time, Roman numerals were still in use and large calculations were executed on the counting board, a form of abacus. These boards were very large, hard to transport, and difficult to use. Extensive training was needed to reach competence, and only a few people could perform the calculations or check them for correctness. Hindu–Arabic numerals were entirely different. Far less equipment was needed to calculate with this system; indeed, ink and paper sufficed. This equipment was easy to transport, and, more important, it was easy to teach and learn. Thus, in a brief period of time the long-established Roman form of calculation was replaced. Although the Hindu–Arabic system limited the need for mental calculation, it helped lay the foundation for further developments in mathematics, especially in areas like number theory, because with the Hindu–Arabic system calculations can be represented on paper and then reexamined later for patterns and structure (Swetz, 1987).

How does this historical case relate to the findings cited above regarding skilled (and not skilled) abacus users? Think again about mental calculation, a cognitive process that research indicates is aided by skill with the abacus. What this history tells us is that the shift from Roman to Hindu–Arabic numerals in the West made mental calculation largely obsolete. It also made it less socially valued because calculating on paper allowed people to demonstrate their solution steps. This suggests that the differential skills of people who do and do not use the abacus may have origins in the mathematical notation shift introduced in the 13th and 14th centuries in Italy. The mathematical skills of abacus experts are consistent with the requirements of the apparatus and the practices their notation system affords, and the mathematical skills of abacus nonexperts who have practice with pencil and paper calculations are consistent with the notation system they use.

The main point from this example for present purposes is that an individual's intellectual history, represented in the tools, symbols, and the thinking they support, are not independent but merged. In other words, they are part of the same problem-solving process, and they reflect the individual's social and cultural history. This example suggests that many of the concepts considered fundamental to human cognition in the domains in which certain artifacts or tools play important roles have not always been in place, at least not in the way they are conceptualized today. Various tools of thought came into being at various points in human history, and these influence contemporary thinking, sometimes in extraordinary ways.

Cognition as a Socially Mediated Process

Finally, activity theory considers intellectual development as a socially mediated process—that is, people have access to the world indirectly rather than directly (Wertsch, del Rio, & Alvarez, 1995). Resources in the social context define and direct the way that information is processed and what is learned. In this view, the formation and development of the mind is inseparable from the social institutional and interactional processes that support the development of this process. That is, material and symbolic tools and social practices mediate the origin and conduct of human behavior, and thereby connect the developing child not only with the world of objects but also with the world of people. In this way, a person's higher mental functioning acquires an organized link to sociohistorically formulated means and operations embodied in cultural tools. This happens as children appropriate these tools through involvement with more experienced cultural members in the specific community in which development occurs.

Cultures develop many types of tools to support the daily activities of people that then mediate intelligent action. These include material tools, like labor-saving devices and forms of technology. Sign and symbol systems, like language, numeracy, and other representational systems, have been developed to represent, manipulate, and communicate ideas. These tools, signs, and symbols provide people with the means to organize and accomplish everyday, practical actions, and their use is passed onto succeeding generations. Through the gradual incorporation of culturally constructed tools and practices over the course of mental development, culture becomes part of each individual's nature.

Organized social practices, or conventions, support this mediational process in that they allow people to share their knowledge with one another. These structures help connect members of a community to each other and to a shared system of meaning. Examples of the connection between cognitive development and cultural ways of organizing and communicating knowledge exist in the developmental literature. Research on *scripts*, which are "outlines" of common, recurrent events (Nelson & Gruendel, 1981), treats the acquisition of culturally organized knowledge as a critical developmental achievement. Research on the development of other pragmatic conventions, such as skill at describing large-scale space (Gauvain & Rogoff, 1989) as if one is being taken on an imagined walk through it (a "mental tour"), also suggests that one important aspect of development is the increasing alignment of knowledge with the conventions of the community in which development occurs.

An intriguing issue is whether these conventional forms influence the process of thinking and its development. There are far less data on this issue. However, a series of studies in an Australian Aboriginal community, the Guugu Yimithirr, is relevant (Levinson, 1996). In this community, the language used to describe spatial location does not rely on relativistic terms, like "left" and "right," but on absolute or fixed directional terms, like "north," "south," "windward," and "upstream." How do these speakers encode spatial information? In one study, objects were positioned on a table in a windowless, nondescript room. Each participant studied these placements. Then he (all the participants were male) was taken to a room with similar furniture but with a different spatial orientation. Once there, the participant was asked to place the same set of objects on a table so as to duplicate the placements in the first room. The participants placed the items in ways that respected the cardinal directions of the original placements—for example, an object placed on the north side of the table was placed on the north side, even though this placement would mean that it would be on the "other side" of an object to an observer using relative position as a guide. Although these results do not specify the cognitive processes underlying this behavior, they suggest that performance on tasks involving spatial cognition involves the coordination of visual and linguistic encoding in ways related to the socially and culturally organized practices of the community.

Especially important for the development of thinking is mediation that occurs during social interaction. In recent years extensive research has been carried out on the influence of social interaction on cognitive development, with much of this research based on Vygotsky's (1978) notion of the zone of the proximal development. Much of this research is described in later chapters. Results generally support the claim that intelligence, especially in the early years, can develop through social experience. This indicates that interaction with social partners, especially more experienced partners, can provide opportunities for cognitive development.

As I noted in the Introduction, dyadic interaction is only one form of social exchange that mediates young children's learning. Parents may influence children's learning via the practical routines they adopt to organize children's behaviors. For instance, research by Munroe and Munroe (1971) in Kenya showed that children's spatial skill was related to the distance they ventured from the home site, but that it was directed distance from home, that is, children's spatial experiences organized by adults to guide children in carrying out activities, such as herding, running errands, and weeding crops in the field, and not children's free-time distance from home, that predicted this skill. Sociocultural influences beyond the dyad also include the network composition of children's social groups (Parke & Bhavnagri, 1989). Beyond the family and peer group, cognitive development is mediated by children's participation in more formal social institutions, especially school. Research across these various aspects of children's social experience suggests that conventions for organizing and conveying knowledge, as well as the social practices through which knowledge is used, mediate cognitive development and are therefore an inherent aspect of thinking.

In summary, activity theory offers an innovative psychological approach to cognitive development through its emphasis on the connection between the individual and the social forces of growth. It describes three features of human social life that may contribute to the development of thinking: organized, meaningful activity; social history; and social and cultural mediation. Together, these outline a starting point for examining the social context as a mechanism of cognitive development. However, activity theory per se is limited for this purpose in several ways.

First, it offers insufficient detail about the range of social processes that contribute to cognitive development and how these processes create change.

Second, the various social partners and social arrangements that contribute to cognitive development in social context are not clearly identified, nor are they linked to specific aspects of growth.

Third, the theory offers inadequate explanation of how the social context may direct or constrain certain aspects of intellectual growth (Cole, 1996). In any particular context, cognitive development involves change in *some* ways of thinking but not in *all* ways of thinking. In addition, an intelligent approach to a particular problem may differ in characteristic ways in different social settings or in different communities. A sociocultural explanation of cognitive development should be able to account for both of these outcomes of psychological development.

Fourth, it is not clear how development contributes to cognitive activity in social context (Miller, 1993). Although this general approach is developmental, the emphasis has primarily been on microgenetic change. Ontogenetic changes are less clearly addressed, even though they are critical to developmental understanding.

Fifth, as in other approaches to cognitive development, there is little consideration of the role that emotions and emotional development play in the process of intellectual growth. Emotions are central to social experience. The emotional context of an activity may play a large role in whatever cognitive developmental outcomes that emerge. Specifying the linkages between emotional experience, social process, and cognitive change is an important part of a social approach to intellectual development.

For all these reasons we must go beyond activity theory to examine the social context as a mechanism of cognitive change. The next section concentrates on the individuals involved in the process of socially organized cognition and its development as a step in this direction. In order to locate cognitive development in social context, it is important to identify who is involved in this process. The developmental literature is replete with studies of how parents and peers influence child development more generally. However, the opportunities and constraints that parents and peers provide for the development of cognitive skill has only recently emerged as an important area of study. To examine this area I borrow a term from anthropology and refer to parents and peers as *agents of cognitive socialization.* These agents are actively involved with children in culturally organized practices that have direct impact on the children's cognitive development. This is because these practices provide the core activities through which children are exposed to and learn about thinking. Although these agents plays different roles in cognitive socialization, they rely on similar processes that appear to be crucial to the development of cognitive skill in social context.

COGNITIVE SOCIALIZATION: WHO'S INVOLVED?

Children have contact with many different people over the course of development. To examine the role of the social world in cognitive development, one must examine how the people that are central to children's lives may contribute to this important developmental process. I concentrate on the two social agents with whom children have the most direct interactional contact: family members and peers. Family members and peers are young children's primary partners in cognitive development.

A third social agent of cognitive development, the social community, will also be touched on in this chapter. Life in the social community, especially formal and informal play and work settings, provides children with opportunities and direction for cognitive development. This is because many of the everyday experiences in which children learn about thinking involve less overt or less didactic social exchange. In this book, these experiences are clustered together and referred to as the *social community of development*. Central to consideration of the social community as an agent of cognitive socialization are the ideas presented earlier in the chapter: the social community is organized or structured, and its members reflect the values and goals of the group. This structure provides opportunities and direction for cognitive development. It is inherent in the activities and institutions in which people are involved and through the tools and resources people use to support intellectual activity. These characteristics of the social community, along with more interpersonal contact, compose the context of human cognitive growth. In later chapters, I will examine these agents of cognitive socialization in relation to specific domains of cognitive development.

The Family

The family has long been recognized as an early and highly influential context for the socialization of all types of skills. Although the family is not the only context in which cognitive skills develop, it is clearly the dominant social context in young children's lives. Children are dependent on the family from early on, and over the years of childhood and through adolescence they are provided with a sustained source of social contact through their families. In addition, family members differ in the expertise, experience, and control they bring to their interactions with children. Both the sustained nature of family life and the asymmetrical relations of family members make the family a powerful and a unique context for cognitive development. Furthermore, the strong emotional bonds that family members have for one another affect the quantity and quality of cognitive transactions in this setting. These bonds may also enhance children's learning and memory in this context, as recent research in developmental and cognitive psychology suggests (Bugental & Goodnow, 1998; Zajonc & Marcus, 1985).

Parental Influence on Cognitive Development

Social interaction in the family is directed toward many goals. A central purpose of these interactions is to provide children with a nurturant and protective environment in which to grow. However, parents also influence children's emerging cognitive skills through the behaviors they encourage and model and through the social and personal experiences they provide for their children both inside and outside the home. Although the behavioral contingencies that parents use, especially rewards and punishments, have been shown to play an influential role in *social* developmental processes, parental influence on *cognitive* development appears to operate differently. The structure that parents provide in face-to-face encounters and in the activities they arrange for children seem to be more effective than behavioral contingencies in helping children learn about and gradually adopt new cognitive skills (Maccoby, 1994).

As I noted in the previous chapter, interactional methods, especially those involving explanation and guided support, that parents use to communicate ideas and ways of thinking to children are especially important in this process. Participation alongside family members in valued community activities also helps children learn about and practice new skills in a supportive, organized, and meaningful context. These methods of cognitive socialization are evident in joint problem solving as a parent explains or demonstrates how to solve a problem by breaking it down into parts and then directing the child's attention and effort toward more manageable subgoals. They also exist at a broader social level as parents organize the household environment and children's daily activities in ways that support and guide their learning and development. For instance, parents play an important role in managing and arranging specific opportunities for children to develop cognitive skills. They frequently determine and monitor children's activities at home, and thereby influence *what* children play and *how* they play. They provide children with afterschool lessons, homework assistance, and technological resources (e.g., computers), to facilitate their learning. They also help arrange children's social activities outside the home, through the activities they encourage for their children and through the neighborhood in which they choose to live. Neighborhood resources, such as the availability of playgrounds, parks, and community centers; neighborhood safety; and the social contacts that children have in the neighborhood also impact opportunities for cognitive growth.

Cognitive development in the family context is not a passive process on either the parents' or the children's parts. Both parents and children actively participate in the psychological dynamics of the family. These dynamics are influenced by characteristics that the participants bring to the interaction. Parents have many characteristics that influence this process, including their personality, beliefs, social history, emotional responsiveness, exercise of control, and expectations concerning child behavior. The contributions that children bring to family interaction are influenced by the child's personality, social history, temperamental qualities, and cognitive skills. And all of these, both the parents' and the child's contributions, are affected by the child's developmental status. Furthermore, the different characteristics that parents and children bring to the family are not independent of one another. Family members are related biologically and socially (Plomin, 1990), and these relations impact the family system in complex and interesting ways.

A social contextual approach to studying the family's role in cognitive development must consider the complexity of family types, the interdependent and bidirectional nature of family relationships, and the existence of the family within the larger sociocultural context. The family system is not an isolated social unit. It is embedded within a larger social system that helps organize its structure and function (Bronfenbrenner, 1986). In recent years, family systems analyses has broadened the scope of what is meant by "family" (Parke & Buriel, 1998). A *family* is no longer defined according to the criteria of the nuclear family. Single-parent families, blended families, and extended families are also functional family units. Cross-cultural analyses have also introduced a range of family types to the study of child development in family context, including very large extended families, clan membership, and polygynous households. Thus, examination of the larger sociocultural context in which the family resides is critical for defining the nature and extent of interactions in which family members engage.

Unique Aspects of Studying Parent–Child Cognitive Interaction

Parental influence on cognitive development has been studied in two ways. In much of the research on this topic, a parent, usually the mother, and a child come to the laboratory and participate together in a cognitive activity. In other research, observations of parent–child cognitive interaction are conducted in more naturalistic settings. Regardless of the setting in which the research is conducted, the participants' prior experiences with one another adds a level of complexity to the analysis. Even in studies in which the cognitive activity is novel to the partners, the partners themselves are not novel to each another. They share an interactional history, and this history may be an important part of what is observed and what children learn in this context. In other words, aspects of the parent–child shared social history may influence the cognitive transaction that emerges in these observations. Thus, consideration of the social history is a necessary part of the analysis, even when research is conducted in the laboratory under controlled conditions (Gauvain & DeMent, 1991).

It is also important to recognize that the activity itself may have been previously practiced or observed in some way by the child. This is particularly the case for observations in more natural settings. Family life is composed of many activities that are similar to one another, that frequently reoccur, and that involve the use of familiar resources or tools around the home. Thus, the child's involvement in these interactions cannot be treated as an isolated behavioral event.

Given these methodological concerns, what research approach may be best suited to examining cognitive development in the family context? Rogoff's (1996) focus on participation may be especially useful in this regard since cognitive development in the family context may be best revealed in the child's changing roles and responsibilities in activities at home. In other words, support and encouragement for cognitive development in the family context involves a reorganization of children's routine activities and participation in these activities in relation to other family members.

Siblings: The Other Piece of the Family Context

Parents are not alone in the family in helping children develop cognitive skills. Siblings are also children's partners in learning. Sibling interaction can provide children with unique learning opportunities. Siblings have frequent and varied types of interaction, ranging from affectionate, helpful, and supportive exchanges to hostile and conflictual interactions. Siblings other than twins have an asymmetry of skill, experience, and control. Together, these factors provide fertile ground for children to observe, practice, and develop cognitive skills.

Although the role that sibling interaction plays in cognitive development is a relatively new area of study, the evidence so far suggests that siblings engage in cognitive interactions differently than do unrelated peers. Azmitia and Hesser (1993) observed young children in a problem-solving situation that also included an older sibling and a same-age friend of the sibling. The researchers found that the younger children observed and imitated the problem-solving behaviors of their older siblings more than they observed or imitated the behaviors of their sibling's friend who was working on the same task right alongside the sibling. The older siblings also helped the younger children (their siblings) more than the unrelated older children did. Finally, the younger siblings solicited more help from their older brothers and sisters than from the other older children.

These observations suggest that the sibling context is a dynamic and bidirectional relationship that can influence cognitive development. This relationship, which has among its many features emotional bonds and familiarity, fosters access to cognitive opportunities. It is important to note that these data also indicate that such interactions can provide growth points for both the older and the younger sibling. The young sibling benefits from exposure to and instruction in more mature or complex skills, as well as from opportunities to request assistance in specific areas of need. The older sibling benefits from instructing and being responsive to the needs of the younger child.

This pattern is reminiscent of research on peer tutoring that has demonstrated that, in many cases, the tutor benefits more from such exchanges than the tutee (Damon, 1984) These benefits emerge from the opportunity to explain one's own understanding to another person who is less knowledgeable or experienced. This opportunity, which can involve articulating a fairly detailed, or perhaps a more simplified, account of a problem or idea, can enhance the older child's learning as crucial features of the task are identified and organized for the explanation. It can also provide practice with perspective taking, in that effective instruction rests on the ability to take the perspective of the listener as a starting point.

Peers

Outside the family the most important influence on cognitive development is a child's peer group. With the child's increasing age, peers assume greater significance. In fact, by middle childhood, the peer group is the main social context of development. Peers play a different role in cognitive development than family members. Interaction with peers is more open and egalitarian than interaction in the family, and these differences can lead to unique opportunities for children's cognitive development.

Over the past two decades the contribution of peer interaction to cognitive development has received increased attention as researchers acknowledge the value of peer experiences on learning and problem solving. Peer interaction facilitates learning because partners often contribute new information, they define and restructure a problem in a way that is familiar, and they generate discussions that can lead to the selection of effective problem-solving strategies (Azmitia & Perlmutter, 1989). Thus, through mutual feedback, evaluation, and debate, peers motivate one another to abandon misconceptions and search for better solutions to problems. This effect has been demonstrated on a range of tasks and domains, including problem solving (Azmitia, 1988), conservation (Doise, Mugny, & Perret-Clermont, 1975), planning (Gauvain & Rogoff, 1989; Radziszewska & Rogoff, 1988), spatial thinking (Mackie, 1983), mathematical thinking (Ellis, Klahr, & Siegler, 1993), and moral reasoning (Kruger, 1992). Much of this research is reviewed later in this book.

Peer Influence in Symmetrical and Asymmetrical Transactions

Both Piaget and Vygotsky considered interaction with peers important for cognitive development. For Piaget (1926), peer interaction is conducive to cognitive development because of the relatively *symmetrical nature of peer relations,* that is, there is relatively little cognitive and social distance between peers. He contrasted these interactions with those characterized by *asymmetry,* that is, those involving partners of different cognitive or social status. The latter were of more interest to Vygotsky.

During interaction involving partners differing in status, that is, interactions in which one child has more power of knowledge than the other, Piaget reasoned, children would be more likely to conform to rules that they do not fully understand or agree with rather than examining the ideas for themselves. When social power is similar, but the peers nevertheless hold different perspectives, Piaget reasoned that the partners would be more likely to participate in and learn from a joint problem-solving process. As discussed in Chapter 2, this set of assumptions led Piaget to be particularly interested in peer conflict and how this may inspire children's cognitive development.

In contrast to Piaget's view of the role of peer interaction in cognitive development, Vygotsky (1978) placed greater emphasis on the role of asymmetrical relationships. He focused on the role of guidance by a person who has achieved a level of expertise beyond that of the child. Thus, much of the research based on Vygotsky's thinking has concentrated on partners of asymmetrical status, for example, adults and children. However, some research does examine peer interaction from a Vygotskian perspective. This research concentrates on peer influence when the peers are asymmetrical in their understanding, examining how peer interaction in such cases may influence the learning that occurs.

The examination of peer cognitive interaction requires sensitivity to several factors, including the children's developmental status, expertise, social skills, social relationship or friendship, and gender (Azmitia & Perlmutter, 1989; Ellis & Gauvain, 1992). These specific aspects of peer interaction, and the role they play in cognitive transactions involving peers, are an important feature of much of the research discussed in the following chapters.

Results from current research on peer interaction and cognitive development suggest that at certain points in development particular forms of social interaction may be more influential than others (Ellis & Gauvain, 1992). Specifically, it appears that learning by observing peers may be especially useful for young children. As children get older, they gain awareness of other people's points of view and learn to negotiate their own and another's perspectives to create understanding (Selman, 1980). For older children, learning by observing peers can still play a role. However, as children get older they engage in more complex tasks that often require much reasoning and integration of thought and action. Such tasks rely heavily on verbal exchange. To communicate understanding on complex tasks requires explanation, often coordinated with some type of demonstration. Thus, most current explanations of the benefits of peer collaboration for children's cognitive development in middle childhood emphasize verbal communication.

Life in the Social Community

Beyond children's social interactional experiences in the family and with peers, life in the community, which Super and Harkness (1986) call the *developmental niche*, also provides children with opportunities for cognitive growth. This occurs through the provision of formal and informal arrangements that organize and direct children's daily experiences, such as schooling and other organized community practices, and through the provision of material and symbolic tools that support learning and thinking. Here, at the outset of this discussion, I must point out that one primary community-based agent of cognitive socialization, schooling, will not be discussed. Schooling has extremely important consequences for cognitive development in many domains of functioning and its impact is apparent in most communities throughout the world. This topic has been the object of extensive study along the very lines of thought presented here (Cole, Sharp, & Lave, 1976; Greenfield & Lave, 1982; Nerlove & Snipper, 1981; Rogoff, 1981; Saxe, 1991; Stevenson, 1982; Stevenson & Stigler, 1992). This book focuses on children's opportunities for cognitive development in the social context more generally, so the cognitive consequences of the specific context of school are not discussed. Interested readers are referred to these sources.

Community influences pertinent to the present discussion are socially organized routines and practices in which children participate and the role of the social partners in organizing and directing children toward these experiences. Less direct social processes, such as children's daily routines, play materials, cultural practices (including the conventions of communication and representation), activity settings (ranging from specific task situations to features of a neighborhood), and social companions, define a substantial portion of the cognitive opportunities that children encounter in their everyday lives.

These experiences may effect cognitive development in a number of ways. They provide children with an introduction to and practice in the activities available in and important to their social community. As a result, they foster the organization and development of particular cognitive skills. Since these activities typically occur in a social setting, they provide children with opportunities to observe more experienced individuals as they engage in these practices, and thereby serve as models for future action. Finally, they provide children with experience using tools and artifacts, both material and symbolic, that are derived from the sociocultural context of development.

CONCLUDING THOUGHTS

The inextricable connection between human biological processes, cultural systems of meaning and action, and their joint passage through time in individual social experience constitutes the landscape of human development. This process benefits both the individual and the community. It serves the individual by guiding his or her developing competencies along valued directions. It serves the community in that it connects generations over time, and connects children and families in communities to one another.

Much of what is currently known about cognitive development was discovered in psychological laboratories in which children worked on cognitive tasks on their own. Whether or how much these findings generalize to children's experience in the everyday social world are open questions. In contrast to the solitary laboratory situation, cognitive development in everyday life is nested within a social world that contains historical, contemporary, and prospective influences. These influences help define and steer its course and they provide opportunities for and impose constraints upon intellectual growth. These opportunities and constraints are built into the social experiences children have, such as social interaction, social institutions, and the cultural tools and artifacts that guide and support intelligent behavior. Together, these help organize the developing mind in ways that are suited to the needs and aspirations of the community in which growth occurs.

Recognition of the embedded, transactional, and complex nature of human cognitive development does not mean that *all* studies must examine *every* aspect of this process. Nor does it mean that cognitive development is solely a social construction. Cognitive development is an active constructive process that involves beings who are evolutionarily predisposed to live and learn in social context with other "like-minded" beings. They are like-minded in terms of both the neurological system available and the social requirements that are in place.

In addition, examination of the role of social experience in the origination of children's thinking does not, in itself, suggest that children have no knowledge from the outset. This is an empirical question that remains to be resolved. But the fact that some knowledge, particularly more basic functions, may be biologically predetermined does not discount the role of the sociocultural context in organizing the expression and use of this knowledge. Furthermore, the argument that social experience plays an instrumental role in the origin and development of higher mental functions does not rule out the idea that more basic mental functions are not biologically provided and/or individually constructed. Some type of skeletal biological structure must chart the course for development in the sociocultural context.

Children's experiences in the family, with peers, and in the community directly affect cognitive development through the opportunities, support, and constraints they exert on children's learning and thinking. These agents help define for children what to think about and how to approach or solve problems. In addition, these social influences operate within a larger cultural context and within a particular historical period. The historical and sociocultural frame of cognitive development is instantiated in the practices, behaviors, tools, and social interactions of a culture and its members. More experienced members are critical in introducing these to children, and in supporting children as they develop and refine these skills in ways aligned with the values, practices, and artifacts of the community. It is in this way that the interpsychological becomes the intrapsychological, and culture is passed across generations. To examine this process in more detail, in Part II of this book I concentrate on cognitive development in social context in several domains of cognitive functioning.

PART II

THE DEVELOPMENT OF SPECIFIC HIGHER MENTAL FUNCTIONS IN SOCIAL CONTEXT

❧ Chapter 4

Acquiring Knowledge: Intersubjectivity, Joint Attention, and Social Referencing

*I*n an early study of mothers and infants, five mother–infant pairs from the Boston area were observed as they engaged in short periods of face-to-face interaction (Brazelton, Koslowski, & Main, 1974). The purpose of this research was to observe what appeared to be a cyclical quality in these interactions. This cycle involved a pattern of looking and not looking, or attention and attention withdrawal, by the mother and the infant. The researchers hoped to determine if this pattern was characteristic of early mother–infant interaction, as well as to find out whether young infants interact with social beings differently than they do with objects.

The observational sessions occurred weekly from when the babies were 4 weeks old until they were 20 weeks of age. At each session, the mother and infant interacted for a brief period of time. Then the infant was observed as he or she looked at an object (a small stuffed animal) that was suspended over the infant's seat. Analysis of the videotapes of these observational sessions revealed that as early as 4 weeks of age, infants pay attention to their mother and an object differently. When interacting with mother, infants exhibited a regular cycle of attention and withdrawal of attention that was much smoother than the pattern of attention the infant directed toward the stuffed toy. In addition, when infants interacted with mother they were attentive longer than when they looked at the stuffed toy. In large part these behaviors resulted from the fact that the mother behaved differently than the object: she moved, she exhibited emotion, and she made direct and responsive contact with the infant. What's more, her behaviors were coordinated with the infant's own behaviors.

Close analysis of the videotapes revealed that mothers used cues from the infants to coordinate their two behavioral streams. Because maternal efforts were responsive to the infant's behavior, the mothers were able to guide the infant's attention in ways that were satisfying to the infant. The infant was not passive in this process and also played an important role. Infants contributed by responding to the mother's efforts and by directing and maintaining their attention in ways that displayed their interests and needs to the mother. This reciprocal process led to a shared focus of attention that was within the infant's grasp. Thus, both infants and adults play important roles in establishing and regulating these early interactions. Although their contributions are not the same, together they create a process of mutual engagement that is based on the infant's emerging attentional skills and the mother's skill at drawing the child into the process. In this way, caregivers provide infants with a supportive context for coordinating their interests and needs with the resources available in the environment. Infants provide fundamental contributions that involve responsiveness, interest, arousal, and engagement. Although rudimentary in form, these behaviors are part of the burgeoning social skills of the human infant and they make the acquisition of knowledge possible.

Despite substantial commonality in the general cyclical patterns of interactions across the five dyads observed by Brazelton and his colleagues, not all the mother–infant pairs in this study interacted in the same way. Some dyads had a smooth interactional flow, and this encouraged infant involvement both concurrently and over time. Infants in these dyads displayed increasingly longer durations of attention during interaction over the course of the several months of study. In other dyads the interaction was less smooth. In these cases the mothers were not as sensitive to their infants' attentional behaviors. Interestingly, the duration of infant attention in these less smooth dyadic interactions did not increase as much over the course of the study as that of infants in dyads who experienced a more coordinated interactional flow.

This research suggests that early social experience, especially with primary caregivers, can influence the development of attention in infancy. The development of attention is important to understand because of its significant role in cognitive development, especially in knowledge acquisition. Attentional capabilities appear early in infancy and are instrumental to all learning. Although much of what develops with regard to attention is a result of basic biological maturation, the organization and use of attentional skills—as this research suggests—is greatly facilitated by social experience. Are the social–cognitive processes involved in the development of attention similar around the world?

Halfway around the globe, in the Pacific Island group called the Marquesas, an ethnographic study of caregiver–infant interaction indicates that there is much cross-cultural similarity in the socialization of attention in infancy. Martini and Kirkpatrick (1981) observed nine infants between the ages of 1½ and 12 months of age and their caregivers. Like the mothers in Boston, mothers in the Marquesas also engaged their infants' attention, and like the Boston mothers they adjusted their behaviors in relation to cues from the infants. Thus, the same type of reciprocity in mother–infant interaction observed by Brazelton and colleagues (1974) among mothers and infants in Boston was evident in mother–infant interaction in the Marquesas.

But an interesting difference was also observed. Like mothers in Boston, Marquesan mothers have much face-to-face contact with their babies during the first 3 to 4 months of the baby's life. In both communities, mothers elicit infant attention during this time by calling the baby's name and identifying features of the baby and mother. Throughout the first year, mother–infant interaction in Western communities continues to include much of this kind of face-to-face contact (Stern, 1977). However, mother–infant interaction on the Marquesas shifts somewhat when the infant reaches about 4½ months of age. The emphasis on face-to-face contact recedes as Marquesan mothers begin to place their babies on their laps with the child facing outward, away from the mother, for much of their time together. Around this same time, mothers' verbalizations also change as they try to direct the infants' attention toward objects and other people in the environment, as in the following utterance made by a caregiver to a 6-month-old: "Baby, where papa? Your papa? . . . It's papa. There, look at papa over there!" (p. 203). Thus, shared visual attention in these mother–infant dyads changed from a primary focus on the dyad itself to one that includes the broader social context of development. This change is supportive of development in this community where children from early on in life have regular caregivers other than their mothers.

Results from these studies indicate that infant socialization of the basic cognitive skill of attention follows a similar course across cultural communities in many ways. Attention is instrumental to learning and acquiring knowledge. More experienced social partners, especially primary caregivers, throughout the world use this emerging cognitive capability in ways that direct the infant's attention to important information and resources in his or her unique developmental context. Thus, it is not surprising that despite much similarity across cultural groups, this process also differs in ways that reflect the practices and values of the social and cultural community in which development occurs.

This chapter is about the social–cognitive processes involved in the development of attention in infancy and early childhood. According to a sociocultural perspective of development, voluntary attention develops through engagement in cultural activities with more experienced community members (Rogoff, 1990; Vygotsky, 1978; Wertsch, 1985). The emphasis is on *voluntary* attention because this involves the active use of cognitive skills to meet personal goals. Since involuntary attention is not under conscious control, it is less sensitive to social input.

Important issues about attention include how it develops, what role experience plays in its development, and what functions it serves in early social, emotional, and intellectual life. Research indicates that the early use and management of attention is influenced substantially by social experience. In fact, shared attention appears to be critical to healthy development. Children with limited ability to engage in shared attention, which is one characteristic of the psychological disturbance autism, have great difficulty engaging with others and thereby learning many important things about the world in which they live (Sigman & Kasari, 1995). This suggests that children come to understand features of the world, including themselves, the thoughts and feelings of others, and the conventional use and value of objects and events, in social situations as more experienced partners direct their attention toward the resources and information in their environment.

To examine the social context in which attention develops, in this chapter I discuss research on three social–cognitive processes that are a fundamental part of the development of attention in young children. These processes are intersubjectivity, joint attention, and social referencing. Before discussing these processes, I offer a brief discussion of the cognitive process of attention, what it is, and how it develops. This is included to familiarize the reader with some of the areas of study in the development of attention from the perspective of individual functioning (for more coverage of this topic, see Weiss & Zelazo, 1991).

This brief review makes clear that much of the early attentional capabilities that infants possess are rooted in basic neurological patterns of growth and maturation. A social approach to this developmental process does not contest this biological base. Rather, it is concerned with a different aspect of this process, namely, the role that the social context plays in supporting, guiding, and organizing the development of attention. This is an important part of human development in cultural context. The attentional system is, in essence, a "gatekeeper" of knowledge acquisition. Because knowledge is intimately tied to the so-

cial and cultural circumstances of development, the social world, especially more experienced community members, play a vital role in guiding the acquisition of knowledge by helping children learn how to
control and use their developing attentional skills. As a result, a complete account of the development of attention requires consideration
of both the biological and the social contributions to this process.

One more comment is in order before I discuss the development
of attention in social context. Because most of the research on this
topic has been conducted with infants, I must mention the general concerns raised by Haith (1997) regarding research on infant cognition.
Haith stresses that in most instances it is difficult, and in some cases impossible, to know for certain what infants understand and are trying to
achieve through their behaviors. Infants' limited communicative skills
prohibit such examination. To try to get around this problem, developmental psychologists can and do design research that isolates and—it is
hoped—discriminates between competing explanations of infant behavior and development. They can also devise theories that avoid over-
attributing cognitive capabilities to infants that cannot be supported
with certainty or that resort to "black box" explanations, that is, an explanation in which some component of the biological system left un-
specified or unstudied is supposed to account for the developmental
process observed. Haith believes that in recent years infant research on
a wide range of cognitive skills has tended to attribute capabilities to infants that have not been clearly demonstrated in research. In particular, he is wary of claims about the innateness of cognitive skills since
such claims tend to be theoretical assumptions that are not subjected to
scientific investigation. He is also concerned about interpretations of
research findings as evidence for high-level cognitive operations without the provision of clear or adequate definitions, observations, and
procedures to support these interpretations. Haith's critique is important to all research involving infants. Although he addressed his comments to the "nonsocial" areas of infant cognition, these concerns also
pertain to early social–cognitive processes. Being mindful of this critique, I have tried to provide conservative interpretations of infant development in this area by concentrating on the behavioral evidence,
pointing out what these behaviors *may* suggest about the early development of attention in social context.

ATTENTION AND ITS DEVELOPMENT

Throughout the world, infants (in fact, all new members of a community) are confronted with the same dilemma: How can I make sense of

all the information I encounter every day? The first step in this sense-making process is directing attention. From early in life attention is used selectively. It is a limited resource that must be used effectively in order to ensure survival. Therefore, some aspects of the environment are attended to closely, others are attended to now and then, and still other aspects are ignored. How are these attentional "choices" made? The word *choice* is used very loosely here. It refers to an active, voluntary direction of attention toward something in the environment. Such a choice need not be reflected upon or even reflectively understood. This stipulation would require more conceptual skill than infants have available. What I mean here is simply attention to one object of focus over another.

Attention is a basic cognitive function that entails the deployment of limited cognitive resources toward specific information in the environment (Gibson & Rader, 1979). Attention develops rapidly over the first years of life. Many basic maturational processes contribute to this development—for example, in the area of visual attention, these include the skills of orienting and tracking. Basic processes such as these involve elaborate neural connections that show rapid development in the first year (Johnson, 1997). In fact, the early and rapid development of attention is not only interesting in its own right, it also provides researchers with a valued way of studying early capabilities in many domains of functioning. The research technique known as *habituation* relies on early attentional skills in that it involves repeating a stimulus to an infant over and over until the infant stops paying attention to it. Infant development in many domains, from language to perception to social recognition, is studied with this attention-based technique.

Developmental research on attention has concentrated on several important changes in the early years, including the control of attention, attentional duration, selective attention, and the relation of attention to other behaviors and competencies. For instance, research on how long children of different ages can sustain their attention to certain objects and actions provides a timetable of the development of attentional control and duration. By 3½ months of age, infants can already control their attention to different sources of information. To study this problem, Haith, Hazen, and Goodman (1988) sat 3½-month-old infants in baby seats and showed each infant a set of 60 stimuli. The stimuli were presented either to the right or the left of center gaze from where the baby sat. Half of the stimuli presented to each baby were shown in alternating sequence, right–left–right, and so on. The remaining 30 stimuli were presented in a random left–right sequence. Infants showed more anticipatory fixations and better reaction times to the predictable alternating sequence than to the random stimuli. In other words, infants detected the alternating pattern, learned it, and then used information from this pattern to regulate their attention to the stimuli. This indicates that, at least for simple visual presentations, even young infants are able to attend to the stimuli and develop or learn expectations consistent with this visual input.

Ruff and Rothbart (1996) characterize the early development of attention as progressing through four major developmental transitions that are regulated by brain maturation. In terms of brain maturation, these transitions involve an initial shift from subcortical control of the visual-looking system early in life to increased cortical control beginning at about 2 months of age. At the end of the first year, with the development of the prefrontal cortex, there is greater involvement of some higher level functions in the attentional system. Between 18 and 24 months, with the development of the lateral prefrontal cortex, there is evidence of some primitive executive functions. Finally, late in the preschool period, the continued maturation of the frontal cortex supports more complex attentional behaviors.

These maturational shifts are evident in changes in attentional behaviors exhibited by children over the first years of life (Ruff & Rothbart, 1996). The first transition in attentional processing occurs between 2 and 3 months of age and is characterized by a shift in scanning abilities away from the external contours of objects toward internal features. Infants also begin to show increased attention toward the novel features of objects during this period. Over the next few months the duration of looking increases and attention seems more investigatory in nature (Gilmore & Johnson, 1995)—that is, infants begin to seek out a focus of attention. From 3 to 9 months of age, infants exhibit increasing control over their attention, especially in selecting objects of interest. The second major transition occurs at about 9 months of age, by which time infants have greater control over looking and its duration and are able to remember past events with only a limited number of cues in the environment to aid remembering. By this age, infants can use attention to solve rudimentary problems like getting toys from behind barriers (Willatts, 1990). For Ruff and Rothbart, these new behaviors suggest a higher system of attention, one based on both physically present information and information available in some form of mental representation, or memory. At 18 to 24 months, a third major change occurs. Now language and other symbolic processes are available and work in relation to the attentional system. A final transition appears later in the preschool years, at which time children are increasingly able to inhibit, or control, their attention. This permits them to carry out more complex tasks, especially those that involve sequencing (or inhibiting) actions. All of these changes are related to and have repercussions for social engagements during the early years, especially during the period of infancy. Table 4.1 summarizes these changes and describes the social–cognitive processes associated with them. These processes are the focus of the discussion below.

Although attention develops rapidly over the early years, young children's attention can be easily distracted. This, too, changes with development and by 3 to 5 years of age children are less distractible (Anderson, Choi, & Lorch, 1987). Interestingly, there is substantial individual variation in distractibility among children at all ages. In fact, distractibility is one of the nine basic categories of temperament, the primary index of individual characteristics and variability in the early years. Research on infant temperament has shown that even in the first year some babies can stare at an object (e.g., a mobile) for a while or play happily with a toy for a period of time. Other babies lose interest rapidly and shift activities often (Rothbart & Bates, 1998). This suggests that despite much commonality in the development of attention, individual differences in attention exist and are associated with other behaviors both concurrently and (some data suggest) over time. For instance, infant attention has been positively linked to levels of play, with infants who display higher levels of attention more likely to engage in complex forms of play for their age (Fenson, Sapper, & Minner, 1974). Also, the ability of preterm infants to sustain attention has been positively associated with later cognitive functioning (Kopp & Vaughn, 1982).

To some degree, individual differences in attention reflect biological differences in the processes that underlie attention, such as autonomic functioning (Porges, 1983). However, individual differences in attention may also be related to environmental factors. Parinello and Ruff (1988) observed the attention of 10-month-old infants to objects during solitary play, as well as the infants' attentional behaviors toward objects when given varying levels of assistance by an adult who directed the child's attention toward the object. The investigators found that infants who had high rates of attention on their own were relatively unaffected in their attentional behaviors when they received assistance from an adult. However, infants who attended relatively little to objects during solitary play were more attentive to objects when they received high levels of assistance from the experimenter than when they received low levels of assistance. This suggests that individual variation in attention not only influences the manner and extent to which children attend to objects, it may also influence children's responsiveness to social input related to attention.

Given the large amount of information available in any situation, the ability to focus on one aspect of the environment and to ignore oth-

TABLE 4.1. Looking, Visual Attention, and Social Engagement in Early Life and Social–Cognitive Processes Associated with These Time Periods

Age	Attentional ability	Socially related attentional behaviors	Social–cognitive processes
0–2 months	Short periods of alertness, organized and selective looking, prefer patterns with large features and high contrast, some tracking, scans edges of stimuli, may fixate on visual stimuli	Interest in faces, some extended looking at faces, may lock on faces or focus on edge area of face	Earliest social interactions[a]
2–3 months	Emergence of orienting or investigative type of attention, longer looking time at specific objects, pattern preferences emerge, more voluntary control of looking, visual engagement/disengagement process smoother	Face-to-face play, makes eye contact, social looking time increases, mutual gaze	Intersubjectivity
3–9 months	Looking time increases, attention more flexible and influenced by experience, rapid disengagement possible, develops expectations based on repetition of simple events, strong preference for novelty, selective visual attention	Attention becomes object-focused in addition to people-focused, increased expectations allow for some control over future looks	Beginning of joint attention to people and objects

(*continued on next page*)

TABLE 4.1. (*continued*)

Age	Attentional ability	Socially related attentional behaviors	Social–cognitive processes
9–12 months	Increased duration of attention, able to look at more distant objects or images, increased control over action, goal-oriented attentional activities emerge	Able to share attention to an object and a person, visual monitoring of faces even at some distance possible, some visual anticipation	Joint attention established
12–18 months	Increased ability to look at complex visual stimuli, increased comprehension of complex visual stimuli	Frequent looks at partner's face, able to follow glances and points of others, able to control attention of others by pointing and vocalizing	Social referencing
18–24 months	Able to use symbolic information (memory of events, language) to direct attention, able to plan and regulate attentional behaviors to meet future goals, self-referential abilities emerge	Social interaction increasingly verbal, language used to direct attention, sense of self develops, ability to regulate attention of self and others	Social referencing includes symbols to direct the attention of self and others

[a]The word *social* is used here in its most rudimentary form. These interactions are "social" in that they involve people; however, the contributions and understanding of the infant and the older person differ substantially. What is particularly interesting in these interactions is that the visual tendencies of the infant, though brief in duration, are sufficiently close to the types of behaviors that people older than neonates use in social interaction to be interpreted as such by infants' interactive partners. This, then, sets the stage for the infant to learn about social interaction by being a participant in the process of social interaction. Thus, as Rogoff (1998) suggests, what is interesting in developmental terms about early attentional abilities and social–cognitive development is not when the infant *begins* social participation, but *how this participation changes* over the early years, with development marked by shifts in the roles, responsibilities, and competencies the infant brings to these interactions.

ers is extremely important for learning. This ability is called *selective attention*. With increasing age, children are more proficient at attending to relevant information in the environment (Schiff & Knopf, 1985). This development reflects, in part, maturational changes in neurological functioning, especially in the region of the frontal cortex (Ridderinkhof & van der Molen, 1995). As children get older, they are more capable of inhibiting their response to distraction, or interference from the environment. Also important to increased skill in selective attention is the fact that with increasing age children use more strategies that regulate their attention, and are more likely to monitor the use of these strategies to reach their goals. For instance, whereas younger children tend to rely on exhaustive search methods when they process information, older children use more selective search strategies (Davidson, 1996). Vurpillot (1968) demonstrated this in a study in which children were shown drawings of two almost identical houses, each containing several rows of decorated windows. The children were asked to determine if the houses were the same or different. Younger children relied on search methods that were haphazard and included attention to the entire array, a process which is overwhelming in terms of the amount of information one needs to process. In contrast, older children compared the windows in a pairwise and systematic fashion. As a result of these selective search strategies, older children were more successful at solving the problem.

In sum, research on the development of attention indicates a very early and rapid pattern of growth. Attentional skills emerge in several ways during infancy and early childhood, including increased control over attention, longer duration of attention, and better use of selective attention to acquire information. Given the pervasive role that social experience plays in early development, it is reasonable to ask how early social experience contributes to this important developmental process.

SOCIAL EXPERIENCE AND EARLY ATTENTIONAL PROCESSES

Early development is greatly influenced by social interaction, especially interactions involving parents and infants. These interactions are reciprocal in that both partners actively contribute to the interaction, and their individual contributions help shape what occurs as well as the outcome of the exchange. Many parent–child interactions, especially in the early years of the child's life, are characterized by the getting and granting of attention. They often involve sensitive responses or scaffolding by the caregiver to the infant's needs and interests. Infants are actively engaged in this process by providing cues to caregivers as to how well their needs and interests are being met. These experiences have both immediate and long-term consequences for the infant. There is evidence that maternal encouragement of infant attention when the infant is 5 months old predicts a significant proportion of the variance in language comprehension and competence at 13 months of age (Tamis-LaMonda & Bornstein, 1989).

The nature of adult–infant interaction changes dramatically over the first year of life as infants' sensorimotor skills increase, as they gain control over their attentional skills, as they develop competence in participating in these social exchanges, and as their interests change. These interactions also change as parents and infants get to know each other better from their shared experiences. Much of this process of mutual understanding occurs in the early months of infancy via face-to-face interactions, when infants and caregivers attend closely to each other's behaviors. The adult's role in these interactions is influenced by the vocal and gestural signals that babies emit, such as those described by Brazelton and colleagues (1974): "The infant assumes a state of attention in which he alternately sends and receives cues. In this state, his arms and legs may pedal slowly, his face alerts, and his eyes dull and then brighten, with fleeting smiles, grimaces, and vocalizations" (p. 56). Signals such as these are interpreted in meaningful ways by adults and are used to organize the adult's response to the infant.

Note that this interpretation can occur *whether or not babies intend their behavior in this way.* In fact, in terms of developmental opportunities, it does not really matter whether infants intend their behaviors in the ways they are interpreted by adults. What matters is that the behaviors serve to initiate an interaction that carries meaning for the adult partner. The meaning of these behaviors is assumed by the caregiver based on a rough guess derived from experience as to what the baby needs or wants. Further communication from the infant that either coincides with or contradicts this interpretation is used to direct subsequent behaviors by the caregiver. In other words, adults modify their behaviors in relation to the baby's behaviors, and use this information to update the initial interpretation. Over time, closer alignment with the baby's needs or interests would be expected to maintain the baby's interest and facilitate or encourage further interaction along this line of meaning. Discordant responses or reactions would not satisfy the infant and would be expected to discourage or curtail the interaction.

The ways in which adults respond to the infant's signals are not uniform across individuals or situations. Rather, they are influenced by many factors, including the individual needs and dispositions of the infant and caregiver, as well as social and cultural frames of reference, like gender-related expectations in the community. Whereas a whimper from a baby boy in a Western community may be interpreted by a parent as whining and overdependency and result in decreased social contact, the same whimper from a baby girl may be interpreted and supported as a need for increased social contact.

To study the infant's contribution to these early social experiences and how this contribution changes in the first year, researchers have observed the play behaviors of parents and infants. Face-to-face play between parents and infants appears when infants are between 2 and 3 months of age. The form of this play is simple. It typically involves the adult talking to the baby and making many overt facial expressions while talking. Despite its simplicity, it does not emerge until the infant is 2 to 3 months of age because this play relies on changes in the infant's behavioral repertoire. Early neonate behaviors are organized around brief periods of wakefulness. Also, neonates exhibit fairly rapid shifts in emotional state. As these behaviors subside in the second month, a different type of social interaction is possible (Thompson, 1998). Also, around this time, the infant begins to produce a broader array of signals that indicate his or her attentional focus. These include orienting behaviors like turning the head and shifting eye gaze. These signals are used by adults as indications of the infant's interest. Adults respond to them in meaningful ways. By the time the infant is 6 to 7 months of age, face-to-face play is replaced by more active forms of play, such as clapping and hiding games. By the end of the first year, locomotion, in the successive forms of crawling, walking, and sometimes running, further broadens the scope of infant social play (Bertenthal & Campos, 1990). Infants are now able to operate more as independent agents in coordinating their attention and the attention of others in ways that help infants meet their goals.

All these forms of play involve mutual engagement by infants and adults in shared, goal-directed activity. However, in order for adults and infants to engage in shared activity, the social partners must establish some form of common ground (Rogoff, 1990). That is, the partners need to have some mutual understanding about each other, such as the fact that they are different agents and that each is doing or trying to do something while they are together. The process of mutual understanding is called *intersubjectivity*. It is essential to communication and its development, and it relies on the basic process of attention.

Intersubjectivity

Intersubjectivity is defined as the mutual understanding that people share during communication (Rommetveit, 1985). Intersubjectivity is essential for communication. It occurs early in infant–caregiver interactions during joint activity when meaning is negotiated by the participants (Rogoff, 1990). Intersubjectivity entails basic principles of communication, including the sensitivity of speakers to the perspective and knowledge of the listeners, a shared focus of attention, and some mutual understanding of how the communication should proceed. Although in early interaction much of the responsibility for establishing intersubjectivity is on the shoulders of the adult, the infant, as we shall see, is at all ages an active agent in this process. The beginnings of intersubjectivity appear very early in infancy. It is through the process of intersubjectivity that attention is socialized; early experience with intersubjectivity helps infants learn about attending to other social beings. This experience helps set the stage for other social processes, especially joint attention and social referencing (discussed below), that build upon and coordinate attentional and social processes in ways that support the acquisition of more complex understanding of the world. Together, these three processes organize infant attention in particular ways, and thereby establish the course of learning and development in the early years.

According to the sociocultural view of development, intersubjectivity creates opportunities for individual cognitive development through the process of social exchange. In other words, through the establishment of and participation in communication that involves mutual understanding (intersubjectivity), children have the opportunity to develop individual cognitive skill. This happens because in order to achieve shared understanding partners must modify their own understanding as they come to understand each other's perspective or point of view. These modifications form the basis of individual cognitive development in social context as they expand children's current understanding beyond what they initially brought to the interaction. The behaviors of adults and infants facilitate this process. For instance, adults may point out connections between new situations and familiar ones, or provide verbal and emotional interpretations of experiences. Infants actively participate as they attend to the information that adults offer and as they provide their own signals that indicate their interest or disinterest.

Much of the early research on the development of intersubjectivity was conducted by Trevarthen (1980a), who was inspired by the films made by Brazelton and his colleagues (1974) of early mother–infant interaction (described at the beginning of this chapter). Trevarthen noted that even 1-month-old infants acted differently when they interacted with their mothers than when they interacted with objects. This suggested to him that any description of human interaction and its role in development could not be reduced to accounts that were nonsocial in nature. This is because during social interaction, relative to non-social interaction with objects, participants must adapt psychologically to one another for the interaction to be sustained.

Trevarthen called interaction between an adult and infant that involves mutual attention to each other *primary intersubjectivity*. The term *primary* refers to the fact that the interaction is interpersonal, concerned with the interactive partners alone, and not with something or someone other than the partners—for example, an object, event, or another person. Interest in the development of primary intersubjectivity led Trevarthen and his colleagues to study early mother–infant interaction. One study explored whether young infants could discriminate social interaction from other forms of social stimuli. To study this issue, Murray and Trevarthen (1985) observed 2- to 3-month-old infants as they viewed a live image of their mothers talking to them over closed-circuit TV. The infants not only attended to these images, they responded animatedly and in a coordinated way in relation to their mothers' behaviors. Later in the session these same videos were replayed for the infants. At this point the researchers observed very different attentional patterns than they had previously seen. After a brief period of watching the replayed image, some infants lost interest and turned away, others became distressed and began to fuss. None of the infants attended to the two videos in the same way. These observations suggest that as early as 2 to 3 months of age infants can distinguish contingent and noncontingent social experiences, that they use their attentional skills in different ways depending upon the nature of the social input, and that they prefer contingent (to noncontingent) social interaction.

Perhaps these results were an artifact of the nature of the stimuli. That is, since both types of social experience were recorded on video, maybe this accounts for the findings. A related study that involved live social interaction addresses this concern. This research was conducted to investigate how infants might react to mothers with depressive symptoms. Cohn and Tronick (1983) asked mothers while interacting with their 3- to 6-month-old infants to adopt an emotionless or emotionally flat expression. When the infants were first exposed to this behavior, they looked at their mothers and tried to elicit a reaction by emitting sounds or moving their bodies. When these efforts failed to change their mothers' expression, the infants became negative or disinterested in their mothers and turned their attention away from them.

Taken together, the data from these two studies suggest that even young infants have some understanding of and expectation concerning the process of social interaction. This understanding may develop over a fairly short period of time after birth or it may be innate. Regardless of the explanation, one thing is quite clear: when normal social interaction does not occur, active engagement by the infant in the interaction stops. When information coming in from the social world is interesting to infants, they maintain their attention to it, at least as long as their developing capabilities allow. This action provides children with the opportunity to learn from others. When information from the social world is not interesting or when it violates whatever expectations infants have about social interaction, infants use their attentional skills to alter or regulate their engagement with the social world. This is fundamentally the same sort of social responsiveness and regulation exhibited by older children and adults. For infants, of course, it is rudimentary in form: the control and duration of attention is limited, and the scope of interest is defined in particular ways. But the point remains that attention to the social world is important and composes a good portion of human experience.

Several other points made in this research need highlighting. The important and active role of the adult is clear. Also evident is the important and active role of the infant. Even at 2 to 3 months of age infants can produce motor expressions, such as orienting the body and the eyes, and emotional responses, such as excitement, irritation, and avoidance, that indicate their attentional focus, and that thereby influence the nature and extent of the social interaction that infants experience. It certainly could be argued that infants' behaviors are actions that are not social in nature but merely interpreted by observers as social. This may be true for some behaviors, like head turning and eye gaze, but the emotional information that accompanies these behaviors, such as excitement or avoidance, are different. For Trevarthen (1980a), emotional expressions such as these are purely social in nature, that is, they have no effect on the physical world other than influencing another human being. Of course, infants need to learn this, and such learning can occur rather quickly. For instance, excitement may initially (i.e., early in life) be formed solely by physiological arousal. However, very quickly the child may learn the association between his or her arousal states and the reactions of others. Finally, although both partners are active in these interactions, their contributions are not symmetrical. Adults, especially early in the child's life, assume more responsibility for initiating and maintaining the interaction. They also have more experience with communication and perspective taking, and they use these skills to support the child's participation.

Although much of the developmental research on primary intersubjectivity has concentrated on its emergence in infancy, intersubjectivity remains central to communication throughout life. Much developmental change occurs in the ways in which children participate in this process beyond infancy. For example, older preschoolers are better able than their younger counterparts to take the perspective of their partner in establishing shared understanding during play. Goncu (1993) observed 3-year-old and 4½-year-old children during periods of pretend play. He found that the older children agreed more with their partners on the roles they each played and on the rules and themes of the play. Older children also maintained the play interaction longer than younger children, and over the course of play older children were able to change the play more readily than younger children. These observations suggest that over the preschool years children's ability to take the perspective of another and use this to establish shared meaning continues to develop.

The origin of intersubjectivity is a topic of much debate (see Schaffer, 1977; Stern, 1985; Trevarthen, 1980b, 1988). For some researchers, the capacity for intersubjectivity is *innate*, that is, infants are born with the ability to share meaning with social partners. For others, intersubjectivity is *learned* through social experience, primarily with adult partners, who initiate this process by assigning meaning to the random behaviors (such as reflexive smiles and involuntary body movements) produced by infants. And for still other researchers, intersubjectivity is a *consequence* of other developmental capacities. For instance, visual perception is largely oriented toward movement, and therefore would include the perception of other people's actions as one category of focus. Even though the origin of intersubjectivity is not known, it is clear that a rudimentary form of intersubjectivity is present early in infancy and that it relies in fundamental ways on the development and control of early attentional capabilities.

One of the interesting questions regarding intersubjectivity is whether the infant's behaviors in these early interactions are intended to communicate with or affect another person. To answer this question requires analysis of the infant's understanding of the meaning inherent in these early encounters. Rogoff's (1990) discussion of this issue is instructive and worth recounting here. According to Rogoff, the notion that someone understands meaning usually includes two parts. First, it includes the idea that an individual can operate on or participate in this understanding in some meaningful way. Infants are clearly capable of this, as their meaningful engagement testifies. Second, it includes the idea that individuals can reflect upon or be aware in some way that they have this understanding. Requiring infants to demonstrate this type of understanding is problematic in that it is beyond their cognitive capabilities. For Rogoff, this dual connotation of the understanding of meaning confounds action (or participation) and reflection and, as a result, obscures the developmental course of intersubjectivity. Like with other processes that develop—for example, strategy development during early to middle childhood—children may be able to participate in actions that rely on the understanding before they are reflectively capable of explaining or demonstrating this understanding to themselves or others. For instance, children use many strategies and use them effectively before they can describe their operation or function or even admit that they have them. Likewise, with intersubjectivity, infants may initially participate in interactions that involve to some degree intersubjective or mutual understanding without being able to reflect or report on this. From experiences such as these, infants develop an understanding of intersubjectivity. This suggests that mature intersubjectivity is an emergent property of social interaction. Infants participate in this process from the outset by providing many cues that get the attention of their caregiver and that then serve as an entry point into these meaningful exchanges. For Rogoff, these may be deliberate behaviors without being at the "top of consciousness," that is, intentional and planned in a reflective sense. Rogoff goes on to suggest that such deliberate moves may characterize many of the behaviors that occur during social interaction, even among adults.

Regardless of the origins of intersubjectivity, infants participate from early on in the first year of life in social encounters that involve shared meaning. These experiences (and the understanding they contain) are primary avenues for learning. They transform over time as children develop and as their social relationships change. An emphasis on early social behaviors as instrumental to learning is consistent with observations by ethologists of the early social tendencies of other mammals (Rogoff, 1990). Reflecting on this finding, Rogoff raises a provocative question about the origin of intersubjectivity in infancy. Perhaps, she writes, more important than identifying the origins of intersubjectivity is understanding why it is that human newborns are less skilled in social behavior than the newborns of many other species. She speculates that this immaturity may provide the flexibility that the human infant needs to learn the social and cultural practices of their unique situation of development.

In sum, intersubjectivity emerges early in infancy as children engage in face-to-face interactions with caregivers. Intersubjectivity involves some sense—though what this "sense" is like for infants is not known—that others are separate from the infant. It also involves some sense—again not well understood—that during social interaction the partners' behaviors operate in relation to one another. Both partners actively engage in this process though their contributions differ, and attention and its development are central to this process. Adults support the development of intersubjectivity by attending to and monitoring the infant's behavior and coordinating their own behaviors with those of the infant. Infants participate as they produce behaviors that communicate their interests and needs through attentional behaviors, such as body orientation, head turning, and eye gaze. Their emotional expressions, like excitement and avoidance, communicate their affective state during the interaction, which provides additional information for the caregiver.

Intersubjectivity is important to development for many reasons. It helps infants learn about the world, as well as learn about the process of social interaction. This process changes over the early years of childhood as children become more able to take the perspective of their partner. Primary intersubjectivity is a stepping-stone to another social–cognitive process that emerges later in the first year of life. Whereas primary intersubjectivity is interpersonal and involves the coordination of the attention of the partners to one another, *secondary intersubjectivity* involves the coordination of three aspects of experience: the infant, the adult, and an object or event of mutual interest. Like primary intersubjectivity, secondary intersubjectivity relies on the development and refinement of attentional skills. An example of secondary intersubjectivity occurs during joint picture-book reading when an adult and infant are both looking at a page in a book. Both exhibit behaviors that specify, support, and encourage their joint object engagement, such as pointing at certain images on the page. Mothers may also scaffold the infant's further development by introducing the names or labels of objects represented on the page. Such behaviors help infants learn the label of the objects depicted as well as the concept of a label (Ninio & Bruner, 1978). Infants may regulate this activity by directing their attention toward certain aspects of the experience. For instance, during the first year, infants may be most interested in the images represented on a page. During the second year, when children show much interest in the way things work, a child may be more interested in turning the page of the book than in looking at what is on the page.

There are two ways in which secondary intersubjectivity uses developing attentional skills to support the acquisition of knowledge. One occurs when an adult and child coordinate and share their attention to an object or event in the world. This is called *joint attention.* The other occurs when infants direct their attention toward an adult in an effort to ascertain information about the environment of which they are uncertain. This is called *social referencing.* Both of these social processes rely on the infant's early attentional skills to facilitate learning and development.

Joint Attention

In 1975, Scaife and Bruner observed young infants to determine if they have the capacity to attend to the same visual target as an adult. In this study, an experimenter first established eye contact with the infant, then the experimenter turned her head 90 degrees and looked for 7 seconds at a target outside the infant's visual range. What did the infants do? Thirty percent of 2-month-old infants turned their heads to follow the experimenter's line of vision. The percentage of children who did this increased steadily with age, such that by the end of the first year of life almost 100% of the infants followed the experimenter's gaze. Since the time this study was conducted, we have learned much more about the developmental course of joint visual attention in infancy, it has been described in much more detail, and related theory has been modified. Nonetheless, this study was a landmark in developmental research because it demonstrated some very important characteristics of the human infant that had, to that point (1975), been largely overlooked. Most importantly, it showed that from very early in life infants use the skills they have available to them to pay attention to the environment and that other social beings play a very important role in this attention-granting process.

In the latter part of the first year, infants display a set of social skills and interactional patterns that collectively point to a new milestone in development called *joint attention*. The ability to participate in joint attention extends beyond the interpersonal focus of primary intersubjectivity. At this time, infants begin to look reliably and flexibly toward the place where adults are looking, they act on objects in ways that adults act on them, and they begin to use active means to direct adult attention to outside entities (Carpenter, Nagell, & Tomasello, 1998). Beyond its impact on the immediate interaction, this important set of changes has been shown to predict later developments in several domains, especially language (Carpenter et al., 1998). Some researchers argue that these skills are also important precursors of social cognition, especially perspective taking and understanding the thoughts and beliefs of others, a topic of much study on the development of theory of mind (Astington, 1993).

What does the process of joint attention involve and how does it develop? Joint attention is the tendency for social partners to focus on a common reference, which may be an object, person, or event, and to monitor one another's attention to this outside entity. It is a social–cognitive process in which three things occur (Tomasello, 1995). First, the social partners know that they are attending to something in common. Second, they monitor each other's attention to the target of mutual interest. And, third, they coordinate their individual efforts during the interaction using their mutual attention as a guide. Interactions involving joint attention help children learn much about the world around them, including what things are important to pay attention to and how these things are valued by others in their community. Because these interactions are set in the context of interpersonal relationships, they are a rich and motivating setting for learning.

Joint attention has been studied primarily with infants and their caregivers because of its emergence between 9 and 15 months of age (Adamson & Bakeman, 1991; Adamson & McArthur, 1995; Tomasello & Farrar, 1986). Most of this research focuses on the infant's visual orientation toward and away from the caregiver and uses this visual orientation as evidence of the sharing and monitoring of attention between social partners. Although joint attention can involve perceptual capacities other than vision, the early development of vision and the ease of assessing attention using visual cues makes this ideal for studying shared attention.

What makes a shared experience joint attention? That is, do all social interactions between infants and their caregivers involve joint attention? In order for an interaction to involve joint attention, attentional monitoring by both partners is crucial. The fact that two people simultaneously focus on the same feature of the environment does not necessarily constitute joint attention. To clarify this issue, Bakeman and Adamson (1984) distinguish *passive joint engagement* from *coordinated joint engagement.* During passive joint engagement, which does not involve attentional monitoring and therefore is not joint attention, the adult and infant are focused on the same object but they do not jointly interact with the object nor do they concern themselves with each other's attention to the object. For example, if a loud noise occurs near a room and both mother and baby turn in the direction of the noise and then turn away, their shared visual focus at the moment of the mutual glance was not joint attention in the sense of a shared awareness or concern with an object of mutual interest. In contrast, coordinated joint engagement occurs when the partners simultaneously attend to the same object and are aware of this shared interest. Their shared experience does not involve the passive sharing of foci, but instead the active construction of attention in relation to the task and activity at hand (Bruner, 1995).

Both adults and children are active participants in this process, though the means by which adults and infants contribute to these interactions differs. Adults monitor the infant's focus of attention and adjust their own gaze to support shared attention. Adults can elicit attention from the infant by either redirecting the child's attentional focus or by following the child's already established attentional focus (Aktar, Dunham, & Dunham, 1991; Tomasello, 1988; Tomasello & Farrar, 1986). Adults' attentional efforts can be expressed in different types of communicative forms, such as visual, verbal, gestural, and motoric forms. Research has shown that infants obtain more benefit in terms of language development when adults respond to cues of interest from the infant, called *attention following*, rather then when adults shift the focus of attention away from what currently interests the infant to some other object of attention, called *attention switching* (Dunham, Dunham, & Curwin, 1993; Tomasello & Farrar, 1986). Certain characteristics of the adult, especially those that may interfere with social responsiveness, can affect the experience of joint attention that infants share with adults. Goldsmith and Rogoff (1995) observed the joint engagement episodes of 18- to 30-month-old infants and their mothers. Some of the mothers were depressed. The researchers found that dyads involving depressed mothers had fewer instances of coordinated joint attention than dyads involving nondepressed mothers. They also found that depressed mothers were more likely to focus increased amounts of attention on the infant when the infant's attention was focused elsewhere. In contrast, nondepressed mothers were more likely to match their attentional focus with that of the infant.

Infants contribute to the process of joint attention through the attentional and emotional skills they have available, as well as by using their emerging social skills. For young infants, eye gaze is an especially important cue during joint attentional episodes. An infant's ability to use his or her gaze to inform his or her partner changes substantially from 6 to 18 months of age (Butterworth, 1995). Whereas 6-month-olds can follow the direction of an adult's eye gaze, they have difficulty determining the precise location of the gaze. By 12 months of age infants can locate visual targets correctly but they do not actively pursue targets outside a set range of view. At 18 months, children are quite competent at directing their gaze, they can even discriminate visual targets that are relatively close in space, and they will search outside their visual view range for a target object. For older infants, other behaviors, like body movements, gestures, and vocalizations, are important. The unique characteristics of the child may affect his or her participation in this process. Sigman and Kasari (1995) compared the joint attentional skills of autistic and normally functioning children. They found that autistic children displayed fewer joint attentional behaviors, such as shared eye gaze, coordinated affective expressions, and duration of attention. The researchers suggest that these differences may reflect differences in the ability of autistic children to monitor the attentional states of others or the ability to coordinate attention and affective information during social interaction. They also suggest that both of these explanations may be true.

Over the first 2 years of life joint attention follows a regular and predictable pattern (Adamson & McArthur, 1995), one that reflects attention changes over this time period (see Table 4.1). Newborns, from birth to 6–8 weeks of age, are able to share attentiveness with their caregiver. However, there is little indication of any sense of shared interest at this point. By 2 months of age the ability to participate in eye-to-eye contact is established. Around 6 to 8 weeks of age, infants begin to display what is called *affective reciprocity* in their face-to-face interactions with caregivers (Stern, 1977). This indicates the beginning of interpersonal engagement, or primary intersubjectivity. Between 2 and 5 months of age, infants have regular and increasing rates of social contact with their primary caregivers. Around this time, infants also have increasing control over their attentional capabilities. Then, at 5 to 6 months of age, infants begin to show interest in objects. Adults support this interest by encouraging and facilitating object exploration. This joint object play can involve simultaneous looking and attending, but before the infant is 9 months of age it is unclear whether the infant knows that the partners are looking at the same thing (Tomasello, 1995). However, by 9 to 10 months of age joint attention emerges as infants show clear signs by referring to or requesting objects socially. Infants do this by visual, gestural, or vocal means, all of which are clearly social acts. Both partners are looking at the object and they are aware of each other looking at the object at the same time. How is it known that infants are aware of this mutuality? At this time infants begin to spontaneously alternate their gaze behavior between the object and the partner during social interactions involving an object (Bakeman & Adamson, 1984). Significantly, the infant does not look at the adult and the object in the same way, which further supports the interpretation that the infant has some awareness of the social components of the activity. The infant expresses affect toward the person but not toward the object (Adamson & Bakeman, 1985). From this point onward, joint attention is increasingly integrated with language, such that by 18 months of age infants will change the direction of their eye gaze to look where the mother is looking when she uses an object label (Baldwin, 1991) and they are able to share attentional focus on absent events with another person by talking about them. Both of these actions indicate increased incorporation of symbolic processing and representations in the organization and regulation of attention. In sum, the first 18 months of life are marked by increased skill at coordinating attention to the social and individual features of an experience (Bakeman & Adamson, 1984). For Adamson and McArthur (1995), this process represents the convergence of interpersonal processes, object exploration, and cultural conventions and symbols as "an object-fascinated infant shares an event with a familiar social partner who is steeped in culture" (p. 211).

This view is supported by cross-cultural research that indicates that the development of joint attention is similar across very different communities (Adamson & Bakeman, 1991). However, cultural variation in the communicative styles and cultural practices with which caregivers establish joint attentional episodes are also evident. For example, among the !Kung San, a hunting–gathering society that resides in Africa, adults neither encourage nor prohibit the infant's exploration of objects (Bakeman, Adamson, Konner, & Barr, 1990). However, if the infant initiates interactions by offering objects to caregivers, joint attention and object exploration follows the same course observed in other communities.

Chavajay and Rogoff (1999) observed the interactions of Guatemalan Mayans and U.S. middle-class mothers and their 12- to 24-month-old children. They found differences in the allocation of attention by children and adults to objects and events in the environment in these two communities. Mayan children and adults were more likely to attend to several events simultaneously, whereas U.S. children and mothers usually attended to one event or object at a time or alternated back and forth between two items in the environment. For example, one 12-month-old Mayan child simultaneously worked at closing a jar lid with the help of an older sibling, whistled on a toy whistle, and watched a passing truck. U.S. children were more likely to play with one toy at a time; if they wanted another toy or to talk to their mother, they would stop their play and do either of these other activities instead. The researchers argued that attention to one or multiple objects or events in the environment at a time may reflect more of a cultural value than attentional capacity. This suggests that the distribution of attentional processes may be an aspect of socialization and thus may reflect to a large degree cultural values and practices.

These studies support the view that caregivers in different social and cultural circumstances are similar in many ways in their efforts to coordinate infants' attention between people and objects. However, this is accomplished in culturally appropriate or meaningful ways. It suggests that joint attention not only reflects maturational changes, but that it is an interactional skill that emerges from joint participation in a shared social context. That is, culture provides a framework that organizes the initiation of joint attentional episodes and also the communicative behaviors that occur in these situations. To find both commonalities and differences in joint attention across cultural communities is not surprising. For Bruner (1995), "Joint attention is not just joint attention, but joint participation in a common culture" (p. 11). Thus, joint attention among cultural members maintains coherence across cultural participants and helps to reformulate culture in each new participant. Here Bruner captures the inherently contextual and developmental nature of the joint attentional process. The social coordination involved in joint attention relies on the integration of minds; features of the context, such as objects, events, and other people; and a shared system of understanding that contains the customs and practices of everyday life about which the mind and features of the world are a part. It is important to note that this description allows for both commonality in the process across cultural communities as well as variability across cultural groups and among individuals within cultures. In other words, by interacting with more skilled partners, children learn about the objects, people, and events in their everyday experience *and* about the symbolic system in their community that is used to label and categorize these experiences.

The processes that support this learning include scaffolding, guided participation, and shared activity. Children learn to attend to objects and events in the world under the guidance of more skilled partners, especially adults. Caregivers provide a supportive structure, or *scaffold,* for infants as they learn to control their attention to the world. The developmental course of joint attention corresponds with the expected role involvement of adults and children functioning in the zone of proximal development (Vygotsky, 1978). For example, a parent may want to share an object with a child. In order to do so, the parent may hold up the object in the infant's range of view and then point at the object while gazing toward it. This helps steer the infant's gaze along the same visual trajectory as that of the parent. To assist the infant even further, the parent may call the child's name and say the object's name aloud: "Joey, look, a ball." In simple, everyday acts such as this, parents help direct the infant's visual attention toward an object, and highlight the appearance and sometimes the name of the object. As children develop, joint attentional episodes undergo fundamental modifications marked by children's active efforts to manage such interactions as well as increases in their repertoire of attentional and communicative behaviors.

Joint attention is important to cognitive development for several reasons. First, joint attention helps direct infant attention toward certain information in the environment. This guidance helps children learn about the world, especially what parts of the world are important for them to pay attention to, as well as how people around the infant feel about this information. Enthusiastic and positive attention affects the child differently than neutral or negative attention. Learning how to direct attention to relevant aspects of a situation is critical to developing competence in all domains of functioning. This is because all types of problems, whether social, emotional, or intellectual, require attention to important problem features in order to be solved.

A second function that joint attention plays in development is communicating to infants that other people can play instrumental roles in identifying objects worthy of their attention. In other words, by attending to objects with another person, infants learn that other people can be helpful for learning about the world. This leads to the understanding of others as intentional agents, which is a chief component of social cognition (Tomasello, 1995).

Joint attention also helps infants learn about the process of language and communication (Bruner, 1975). Joint attention is especially important to the development of referential communication skills as children learn how to label objects, events, and people in ways that are conventional in their language. Joint reference to objects, events, and other people also provides opportunities for children to participate in the process of negotiating meaning as the partners interpret information in the environment or determine what is important about it. In this way joint attention is instrumental to the development of language (Bruner, 1975). Finally, joint attention allows children and adults to share experiences with one another. This has cognitive consequences, like learning the names and importance of objects. It also contains emotional messages about the partner's relationship and helps construct their unique history of shared experience.

As is true of primary intersubjectivity, the origin of joint attention is debated. Differing views on this question reflect the range of stands represented in the more general nature–nurture debate (Dunham & Moore, 1995). Certain maturational skills, such as gaze behavior, clearly need to be in place for this social process to appear. The extent to which experience, especially social experience, is critical in refining, aligning, and coordinating attentional behaviors, like head turning and orienting, that are involved in the joint attention process is less clear. For some researchers, especially Tomasello (1995), the development of joint attention also relies on the emergence of social skills that make this process possible, such as communicative gestures and imitation.

Social Referencing

The third process relevant to knowledge acquisition in social context that emerges in the period of infancy is social referencing. *Social referencing* is the process by which an individual looks to someone else for information about how to respond to, think about, or feel about an object, another person, or an event in the environment (Campos & Stenberg, 1981; Feinman, 1982). Social referencing involves joint attention because a shared focus of interest between the individuals is involved. However, the concept of social referencing stretches beyond joint attention by including the idea that the social partner, typically an adult, informs the child in emotional and sometimes instrumental ways about the object or event of focus.

Social referencing in infancy appears late in the first year of life. When an unfamiliar object or uncertain event occurs in the infant's presence, the infant 9 months of age or younger will stare at it. Although the infant may take some form of action in relation to the object or the event, the infant will not look to others who are present for guidance in this regard. At about 9–10 months of age this behavior begins to take a dramatic turn: now, in such circumstances, infants begin to look at or refer to others who are present. These looks precede the infant taking any action in relation to the object or event. What's more, the way in which the child acts in this situation is influenced by the information he or she obtains from the other person.

This process has typically been studied in a laboratory situation in which a child and a caregiver are present in a room when an unfamiliar object appears or an uncertain event occurs. The unfamiliar stimuli used in research have included an unusual or novel toy, such as a robot that makes songlike sounds or a remote-control toy spider; a situation of uncertainty, like placing the infant on the edge of the precipice or "dropoff" in the visual cliff apparatus used to study infant depth perception; or an unfamiliar adult, somewhat like the child–parent–stranger episode in the "Strange Situation" procedure used to study parent–infant attachment. In order to investigate whether children's reactions to such stimuli are affected by the social context of the situation, the adult in the experiment, who may be either a parent or an experimenter, is instructed to express a specific emotional reaction, such as happiness, fear, or disgust, when the object or event appears. This serves as the independent variable. The dependent variable is the infant's actions toward the stimulus following exposure to the adult's reaction.

For example, in Klinnert's (1984) study, 12- and 18-month-old infants and their mothers were presented with three novel toys. The mothers were trained beforehand to show either a smiling, a fearful, or a neutral expression when a toy appeared. Klinnert found, first of all, that most of the infants looked at the mothers after each of the toys appeared. Results also showed that when the mother's face expressed happiness, infants tended to move away from mother and toward the toy. The mother's positive expression apparently encouraged more active object exploration. However, when the mother's face expressed fear, infants moved toward mother and away from the toy. The

mother's negative expression apparently discouraged further exploration of the object. A neutral expression resulted in mixed or intermediate responses. Results from this research and the many other studies
like it indicate that the emotional response that adults display toward
new or uncertain situations in an infant's presence is influential in
guiding the infant's subsequent actions in that situation (Saarni,
Mumme, & Campos, 1998). Research also makes clear that infants actively seek this information and then use it to organize their own behavior.

Thus, by the end of the first year of life, infants regulate their own
behavior in certain circumstances in relation to the socioemotional
context of the experience. Infants more readily accept and approach
objects, other people, and situations when they detect positive messages from others about these aspects of the environment (Feinman,
Roberts, Hsich, Sawyer, & Swanson, 1992). When negative messages
are detected, unfamiliar objects, people, and events are treated more
cautiously or avoided all together. One study (Barrett, 1985, cited in
Feinman et al., 1992) found that when infants were exposed to incon-
sistent emotional messages (e.g., a smiling face accompanied by negative gestures) about an object, the infants looked at the adult more and
were more likely to be ambivalent toward the toy than when consistent
messages were expressed.

What skills do infants need in order for social referencing to occur? The answer to this question describes important developments in
the cognitive, especially attentional, and social domains over the first
year that underlie and support this process. First, the infant needs to be
attentive to the environment and to new information or experiences
present in the environment. This reflects changes in the perceptual and
attentional systems, especially increased sensitivity to visual information and discrepancies including patterned information from the voice
and face (Campos & Stenberg, 1981). Second, the infant needs to attend to the other person present, especially to the emotional messages
being communicated. Implicit here is some recognition of other beings
as separate from the infant and different from inanimate objects.
Third, the infant needs to understand the content of the other person's
emotional message. This includes distinguishing one type of message
from another, identifying what a specific message means, and being
able to respond appropriately. Research indicates that infants can do
this as early as 6 months of age for basic emotions such as happiness,
fear, and disgust (Walker-Andrews, 1997). Fourth, the infant must be in
what Feinman and colleagues (1992) refer to as "an appraisal mode."
This means that the infant must not only be ready to detect the emotional messages of another, he or she must also be ready to process this

information and to construct some understanding of the event from this message that is useful for guiding action. This ability seems present in some rudimentary form at about 9 months of age. Finally, the infant must be able to identify the specific referent of the emotional message, a skill that appears by the end of the first year. This ability was demonstrated in a recent study by Repacholi (1998) who investigated whether infants could use attentional cues to identify the specific referent of another person's emotional experience. An experimenter referred to two different objects that were hidden in boxes in an infant's presence. Each object received the same amount of attention from the experimenter, but each was associated with a unique emotional message. The experimenter would open each box, look inside, and then display either happiness or disgust in response to seeing the contents of the box. The infants could not see the objects in the boxes. Infants as young as 14 months of age were able to correctly identify the specific target of the emotional expression as the object inside the box and not the box itself. This was evident in the infants' behaviors: the infants were more likely to put their hands into the box associated with the happy expression, but they did not differ in their touching of the two boxes. These results suggest that infants seek cues about the specific object of the adult's focus and are not just looking in the direction of the adult's gaze and using this to inform them in a more general way.

Information provided by the social partner during social referencing can be emotional, instrumental, or both. In truth, most of the research on social referencing has emphasized the emotional content of this type of exchange. In terms of emotional information, what transpires is that the more experienced individual, usually a caregiver, conveys to the infant an evaluation or appraisal of the object or event of shared focus. The infant then uses this information in some way to organize his or her subsequent action in the situation. So far, this description makes the process sound unidirectional, with information flowing from the more to the less experienced participant as a direct form of imitation or instruction. However, it is important to stress that the infant actually plays an active, constructive role in this process (Rogoff, Mistry, Radziszewska, & Germond, 1992). This is evident in several ways. The infant needs to perceive the object or event (the referent) in the environment and attend to it. The infant needs to seek further information about this referent from someone else in the setting, usually a familiar person. Finally, the information received socially is used in some way to guide the infant's subsequent action in relation to the object of interest. This requires combining an emotional message from another with the infant's own emerging understanding and appraisal of the situation and translating these into actions or instrumental behaviors toward the object or event. In other words, infants construct understanding of the situation that then guides their behavior. This understanding is informed, but not dictated by, the social information available in the situation.

Evidence of the infant's active or constructive contribution to this process includes the fact that the infant does not simply imitate the emotional information he or she detects. Rather, this information is used to guide the instrumental actions of the infant, such as approach or avoidance, in relation to the situation. Since these actions are not modeled by the other person, they are not available for imitation. Further evidence of the infant's active contribution to this process appears in efforts by infants to negotiate or challenge the interpretation of the event offered by the adult. For example, Walden and Ogan (1988) observed that 14- to 22-month-old infants would sometimes touch a toy about which they had received fearful messages from their mothers. However, these touches were accompanied by a smile by the infant directed toward mother, suggesting some challenge or disagreement with the mother's message.

Several aspects of social referencing have been studied rather extensively to clarify this process. One of these aspects concerns whether situational uncertainty or ambiguity is essential for social referencing to occur. Research indicates that social referencing is most likely to occur in situations of uncertainty, but that it can occur in all types of situations (Klinnert, Emde, Butterfield, & Campos, 1986). This suggests that socially derived information may impact many aspects of children's learning, even cases in which children already know something about the situation. This was demonstrated by Rosen, Adamson, and Bakeman (1992) who studied responses to a situation by two groups of infants: those who looked at their mothers before they reacted to a novel object and those who looked at their mothers after they produced an initial reaction to the novel object. Both groups are important to study, though most research up to this point had concentrated on infants who seek adult information before reacting to the situation. About half the infants in the Rosen and colleagues study looked at the mother before reacting to the object, and about half reacted to the toy and then looked at mother. Very few infants reacted to the toy and never looked at mother. Comparisons of the first two groups of infants indicated that the mothers' emotional messages were equally effective in guiding the infants' behaviors over the session regardless of when the infant's initial look took place. The authors use this evidence to support the view that social resources are used by infants as an ongoing source of information about situations, even when infants have their own initial reaction to the situation.

Other research has examined the identity of the referee—specifically whether or not it must be a known or trusted person. Results show that, all things being equal, infants are more responsive to messages from a parent than from a stranger (Zarbatany & Lamb, 1985), and that mothers and fathers are equally effective as sources of reference in these situations (Hirschberg & Svejda, 1990). However, if a parent is not providing helpful information or appears puzzled, a stranger who is confident in conveying emotional messages about the situation will be used as a source of reference over the parent. For example, Klinnert and colleagues (1986) asked mothers in some situations to act puzzled. In these cases, infants looked at the stranger who was present more than at mothers.

Taken together, these observations suggest that from early in life other people play a fundamental role in knowledge acquisition. Infants attend to such messages from others—in fact, they actively pursue them—and they use this information to organize their further interactions with the world. This, then, helps shape further learning as some situations are explored in more depth and others are not. Because infants play an active role in seeking, negotiating, and using this information, social referencing suggests a different view of development than approaches that consider interaction with other people as merely a passive form of social stimulation. In contrast, social referencing is an active process of social construction, one that is consistent with Vygotsky's (1978) emphasis on the important and dynamic role that social experience plays in individual mental growth. Although social referencing makes its initial appearance in the latter part of the first year, it remains important throughout life as people interact and use each other to devise meaning and interpretation for experience (Feinman, 1992). The beginning of this process in infancy is an important developmental piece of the lifelong human ability to engage in reciprocal intentional communication (Bretherton, 1992).

Thus, social referencing is a part of the social context of knowledge acquisition that is used reliably, flexibly, and frequently by infants and toddlers (Adamson & McArthur, 1995). However, it is important to stress, as Bretherton (1992) does, that the information provided by social agents may not always be helpful. In fact, studies that investigate social referencing demonstrate this very point by showing that infants will steer away from a perfectly acceptable toy when an adult displays a negative expression. As in research on the zone of proximal development (Goodnow, 1987), research on social referencing has tended to emphasize the beneficial aspects of these social cognitive experiences. It is important to remember that these processes can have both positive and negative outcomes, and that research on the range of consequences of the social context of knowledge acquisition is needed, especially research on the early years of life when children are heavily invested in this process.

The origin of social referencing is debated along the same nature versus nurture lines discussed in the sections on intersubjectivity and joint attention. That is, some argue that this process follows a maturational course and others contend that over the first year infants have sufficient experience with others, especially primary caregivers, to discover that social agents can be used reliably as sources of information about the world (Gewirtz & Pelaez-Nogueras, 1992). As in the other areas of study discussed in this chapter, the answer to this debate is likely to be that both nature and nurture contribute. There is less debate about the developmental functions that social referencing serves (Feinman, 1992). Several of these functions are directly related to emotional development; these are discussed in detail in several sources (Feinman, 1992; Saarni et al., 1998). Our concern is the contribution that social referencing makes to cognitive development.

First, in the cognitive domain, social referencing is a central process by which infants construct understanding about the world. Furthermore, through social referencing infants appropriate information about the world that contains the knowledge (and biases) of more mature persons. This creates a basis of shared meaning, which is supported by the fact that during social referencing infants almost always refer to individuals with more experience than the infant (Adamson & McArthur, 1995). The infant uses this information to construct his or her own understanding of reality. Thus, by referring to more experienced individuals, especially in new or unusual situations, infants have the opportunity to learn the knowledge accumulated by members of their community instantiated in the behaviors of an experienced individual. This asymmetry of knowledge, according to Adamson and McArthur (1995), positions the infant as a cultural apprentice. In this way, the social world plays a key role in mediating knowledge acquisition from very early in a child's life, and helps ensure the survival of the infant now and the community in the future. This process has consequences beyond the individual. By participating in this process, infants learn the conventional or socially shared interpretations of situations. That is, they are enculturated into the understanding of the family and the community in which they live (Thompson, 1998). Because this is an active, constructive process, it provides opportunities for both continuity and change for the cultural community.

Second, social referencing provides infants with specific information about a situation. This information, which can be either emotional or instrumental (or both) in form, helps infants learn about the immediate environment and how to manage or cope with it. The emotional information is evaluative in nature, and cues the infant as to whether something is likely to be pleasurable or not. Instrumental information includes ways of dealing with the situation, especially by encouraging or discouraging further exploration. The value of this information is evident in the fact that infants do not refer to social agents who cannot be relied upon for useful information.

Currently more is known about the role or function that social referencing has in development than about how this process works (Feinman, 1992). It is clear that the process relies on the information-gathering skills of the infant, and that these skills are coordinated with motivation by the infant to seek knowledge, especially certain types of knowledge, about the world. However, how the perceptual, attentional, and motivational systems work together in this process is not understood. In addition, the role that language, including productive and receptive language and nonverbal communication, plays in this process is not well specified. Also, little is known about how the social messages about the world that infants receive are interpreted or transformed into knowledge. This is particularly puzzling when one considers how brief these interactions or exchanges are. And, finally, how does this knowledge get translated into action? The bulk of research on this topic has been on the emotional aspects of social referencing and how this contributes to emotional development. However, the role that social referencing plays in cognitive development, specifically in organizing the content of the knowledge base, the actions that accompany this knowledge, and the process of knowledge acquisition throughout life, is significant and merits further study.

What is known for certain is that social referencing plays a critical role in knowledge acquisition from late in the first year of life, and that it continues to play an important role throughout life. This role changes with development, with the young (or inexperienced) more likely to seek this type of assistance than more experienced individuals. This process is especially pronounced early in development. Research has found a fairly consistent pattern of social referencing and its effects well into the fourth year of life. There are some developmental differences even during this period, however. For example, in the Walden and Ogan (1988) research mentioned above, infants between 10 and 13 months of age were observed to interact with toys in ways consistent with the emotional expressions of adults. However, between 14 and 22 months of age infants show what the researchers refer to as "rebellion" in their behaviors by sometimes touching the toy associated with a fearful message more than the toy associated with a happy message. Furthermore, when the infants touched the toy associated with a fearful message they would smile at their mothers. The researchers believe that this may represent an early bid at negotiating the meaning of the situation with the caregiver. These observations suggest that very soon after children begin to participate in social referencing, they begin to negotiate the meaning of the situation that is offered by others. This is further support for the claim that children actively construct knowledge during social referencing.

Despite general developmental trends in children's participation in the process of social referencing, there is also individual variation at each age in how social information is sought and the degree to which it affects child behavior. Child characteristics, like temperament, and parent–child characteristics, like attachment, may play a role, although not all studies show evidence of this linkage (see Feinman et al., 1992). Autistic children rarely seek information from others in these types of situations, and when they do look at others their glances are briefer than those of normal children (Sigman & Kasari, 1995). There is some evidence that child gender may play a role in the emotional messages that adults convey and the reactions that children have to these messages. Rosen and colleagues (1992) found that child gender did not relate to the number of times infants sought information from mother. However, they observed that fearful messages to girls were significantly less intense than fearful messages to boys. This may reflect different sensitivities or responsiveness to mother's emotional messages by girls versus boys or different socialization efforts extended toward girls versus boys (or both of these explanations). These different messages are especially interesting in their relation to the children's toy-related behaviors in this study. The distance that girls, but not boys, had from the toys was modulated by the mother's emotional expression. Girls stayed closer to the toy than mother in the happy message condition. In the fearful condition, girls were equidistant between the toy and mother. In contrast, boys stayed closer to the toy than to mother in both conditions. Finally, other factors, such as parenting styles, expectations for conformity in a family or a community, and sensitivity to nonverbal messages in individuals or across communities, makes social referencing an especially good area for further study, particularly in relation to family and cultural practices. The importance of this direction of study is underscored by observations made by Thompson and his colleagues (cited in Thompson, 1998) that adults are aware of their influence on children in this regard and deliberately present salient emotional information to guide their children's actions.

CONCLUDING THOUGHTS

This chapter discusses early cognitive development in social context by examining three social–cognitive processes—intersubjectivity, joint attention, and social referencing—that are tied to the infant's emerging attentional capabilities in the early years. These processes play important roles in the content and process of knowledge acquisition in the first years of life. They are part of a rapidly emerging social, cognitive, and emotional system during infancy that serves many purposes and establishes a lifelong pattern of learning, communication, and social relations (Tomasello, 1995). Furthermore, these processes are developmentally organized—that is, they build upon each other. They also help set the stage for a way or process of learning that is essential to further development. These three social–cognitive processes contain within them the knowledge of the community in which development occurs, represented in the assistance of more experienced community members, especially primary caregivers. The affectional bonds between young children and their caregivers serve to strengthen these processes of knowledge acquisition. Children are active agents in processes of knowledge acquisition, and this ensures both continuity and change in development. The potential for continuity and change through these processes provides adaptive benefits for both the individual and the community in terms of what is known about the world and how this knowledge is interpreted to guide action.

Although this chapter emphasizes the rudimentary or early stages of shared meaning and its active construction in infancy, these processes are part of knowledge acquisition throughout life. The following chapters discuss cognitive changes that are also social in nature and that have, implicit within them, the three fundamental social–cognitive processes for knowledge acquisition discussed in this chapter. Because these processes are already part of the child's repertoire by the end of infancy, they are instrumental in supporting development in many areas of cognition.

Chapter 5

Remembering: The Social Construction of the Past

Midway through the family's holiday dinner 5-year-old Molly was asked to tell everyone about her first day at school. She hesitated, and then said it was fun. After a long pause, during which it became clear that she was done, she was asked for more details: "Who's your teacher?," "Is she nice?," "Did anything special happen that day?," "Did you have a snack? A nap?" A lively exchange went on for close to half an hour, by the end of which everyone had learned quite a bit about Molly's first day at school. Her grandmother remarked that it sounded like a great day, and Molly was pleased both with her first day at school and with her report about it to her family. In fact, when Molly's mother thanked her for telling everyone about her day, Molly exclaimed, "Yes, and I did it all by myself!"

This type of comment is fairly common among young children. What happened in this interaction was that an individual's memory was prodded and probed—essentially "excavated"—by others until a satisfactory story emerged. This type of interaction is a reminder that memory and remembering are not solely internal processes. Memory is often a social process, one that involves mutual efforts to recount the past. This process begins very early in life. Parents and children are involved in talking about the past almost as soon as a child learns to speak (Eisenberg, 1985).

Many features of social interaction aided Molly in her remembering. The adults used the conventional routines of kindergarten as a guide for formulating questions. Other lures, such as asking about events of personal interest or significance, also occurred. Recall that all that Molly remembered at the outset, or at least reported remembering, was that it was a good day. Coaxing, framing, and interest from the family, and cooperation and collaboration from Molly, brought the memory into being. This process is called *social construction*. According to Halbwachs (1980), all memory is shaped by the social environment and derives from social interaction. In other words, the social world is a constituent factor in the construction of memory. Notice that the word *construction* is used here. Even though we often think of memories as something akin to stored facts, like library volumes, in actuality memories are actively constructed pieces of knowledge (Bartlett, 1932; Bransford & Franks, 1972). People neither encode nor recall events verbatim, exactly as they happened. They "construct" a memory of the event, and this construction is influenced by many factors including the social and cultural context of remembering.

The idea that memory is a social process is not new to psychology. It was of central concern in Bartlett's (1932) early studies of memory. According to Bartlett, societies provide individuals with schemas that affect how and what they remember. A *schema* is a knowledge structure that has been acquired from prior experience. Schemas influence the way people encode, interpret, and store new information.

It is well established that schemas aid individual memory and its development (Mandler, 1984). What is normal, typical, or expected, that is, reflects preexisting knowledge or schemas, is remembered better than that which is unusual or unexpected. However, according to Shotter (1990), the main function of schemas is not to enhance individual storage. Rather, schemas serve a social function, one that supports the processing of information and the sharing of knowledge and memories within a culture. This, in turn, ensures continuity over time and people. Implicit in this view is the idea that the development of knowledge or memory entails the appropriation of schemas across generations that then work to connect children to their own unique history and to the history of their cultural community. Socialization provides children with interpretive schemas, or frames that assign meaning to events (Costanzo, 1991). In other words, through social experience children acquire understanding of the world and of themselves, and this becomes the basis of their knowledge system, their memory. Social experience also provides children with opportunities to learn and to practice ways of remembering. Not all knowledge is remembered effortlessly. Sometimes strategies are needed to encode, store, and retrieve information. Although there is no doubt that children develop memory strategies, it is not well understood how these memory strategies develop or why children develop some strategies and not others.

This chapter is about memory. It begins with a brief discussion of what memory is and why it is important. Several excellent sources describe the development of memory from the perspective of individual performance and change; the reader is referred to these for further discussion of this process (Fivush & Hudson, 1990; Gathercole, 1998; Kail, 1991; Schneider & Bjorkland, 1998; Schneider & Pressley, 1989). Because my focus is on the social contributions and social character of the development of memory, I concentrate on the role of social experience in this development. I examine how social experience influences both the content and process of memory. Examination of the development of memory in social context raises many provocative questions about the nature of memory itself, including Where does social memory stop and individual memory begin? As you will see, this is not any easy question to answer.

WHAT IS MEMORY AND WHY IS IT IMPORTANT?

No other area of cognitive development is studied more than memory. Research on the development of memory has a long history in the field of psychology: the earliest studies of memory development appeared in the late 1800s, shortly after the birth of psychology itself (Schneider & Pressley, 1997). Nelson (1996) considers memory the primary form of mental representation from which all other forms, including concepts, categories, schemes, imagination, and plans, are derived. This accords with Vygotsky's view that "memory in early childhood is one of the central psychological functions upon which all the other functions are built" (1978, p. 50). Although it is true that only a subset of developmental studies explicitly address issues involving memory, if one looks deeper, it is clear that memory is part of almost all mental activity and therefore part of most developmental research. This is so because everything we know involves memory. In fact, the terms *memory* and *knowledge* are interchangeable. Acts of memory range from rapid-fire basic processes, like face and word recognition, to recall of complex knowledge systems and events, such as the rules of chess and how a family coped with the Great Depression.

Memory is a multifaceted process, that is, there are several different types of memory and these have different neurological bases (Schneider & Bjorkland, 1998). Some types of memory are influenced substantially by experiential factors, while other types are less influenced. Most models of memory consider this process to be composed of multiple steps of processing. Figure 5.1 provides a diagram of these steps. The initial step involves the processing of sensory input, which is referred to as *sensory register*. This process is brief, lasting 1 to 4 seconds, during which the sensory system either retains information for further processing or not. If retained, the information is held in short-term, or working, memory, which is the conscious area of memory. Short-term memory has a limited storage capacity of about seven items of information (Miller, 1956). Information retained longer in memory is transferred to long-term memory, or storage, which potentially has boundless capacity and no temporal limitations. Long-term memory contains a vast array of information, including all the world knowledge and facts a person possesses (called *semantic memory*) and memory for events (called *episodic memory*). Much of episodic memory is autobiographical in nature and includes memories of important events or experiences that have happened to an individual. Much of the discussion below on children's memory in the early years of childhood focuses on the emergence of autobiographical memory.

The act of remembering can be either intentional or unintentional. Much of everyday experience with memory involves unintentional forms of acquisition, retention, and retrieval. It is rarely necessary to exert intentional effort to recall language, such as vocabulary and speech forms; behavioral routines and procedures; and personal experiences. This kind of information is simply encoded, retained, and recalled when needed. In contrast, intentional memory, which is also called *explicit memory*, requires overt effort during storage or recall. Much of the developmental research on intentional remembering concentrates on *strategies*—for example, organization, rehearsal, and elaboration—that aid storage and retrieval. Over the years of middle childhood, children's skill at using strategies, like organizing items semantically and storing information in meaningful categories, increases. While the reasons underlying these changes remain unclear, the evidence discussed below suggests that some of this change may be due to social experience.

As in all areas of cognitive development, biological and social processes contribute to the growth of memory. Some areas of memory de-

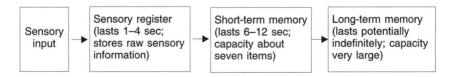

FIGURE 5.1. Multiple steps involved in memory processing.

velopment are more influenced than others by maturational processes. However, even these show some changes in the course of development as a result of social experience. *Processing speed* is the rate with which incoming information is processed mentally. Between early childhood and adolescence, speed of processing increases (Kail, 1991). This increase is thought to result from neural changes associated with age, especially increased mylenization of the neurons and the elimination or pruning of unnecessary neural connections, both of which contribute to increased efficiency in processing information. There is also some evidence that domain-specific expertise may increase the speed with which children process information in that domain (Roth, 1983). This suggests that experience contributes to this basic memory function. A second area of memory change that is largely maturationally based is *memory capacity,* or the amount of information that can be held in working memory. In general, the amount of information that children can remember increases linearly with age. However, once again, evidence suggests that domain expertise can influence children's memory capacity (Chi, 1978). Thus, even in two areas of memory development that are largely regulated by maturational processes, experiences provided by the social and cultural context of development play an important role.

EARLY EVIDENCE OF REMEMBERING

Some of the earliest evidence of memory in childhood appears in neonates, who at 1 week of age can recognize their own mother's smell. To discover this, Macfarlane (1975) used a preferential looking task in which he positioned an infant between two nursing pads, one used by his mother and one used by another nursing mother. When the infants were a few days old, no preference was evident. However, by 1 week of age, infants turned in the direction of their own mother's nursing pad, indicating that they recognized her unique odor.

Some research suggests that babies may even have recognition memory while they are still in utero. DeCasper and Spence (1986) asked pregnant women in the last 1½ months of pregnancy to read aloud twice a day a passage from the children's book *The Cat in the Hat*. After birth, when the babies were 2–3 days old, they were given the opportunity to listen either to this same passage or to a reading by the mother of a passage from another children's story. Babies sucked on a pacifier while they listened to an audio tape recording of the stories. The rate with which the baby sucked on the pacifier controlled which passage the baby heard. If the baby sucked at one rate, one passage was audible. However, if he or she switched the rate, the other passage was audible. For some babies, the switch from the familiar to the new passage required increased sucking, and for some babies it required decreased sucking. Regardless of whether the babies had to increase or decrease their rate of sucking, infants modified their rate in the direction that produced the familiar passage from *The Cat in the Hat*. In order to do this, auditory recognition of maternal intonation was required.

Although the results of studies such as these cannot tell us what is in the baby's head at the time these behaviors were produced, we can nevertheless conclude that some form of memory was involved. Whether this is the same memory process that adults use when they remember sounds and smells is unknown. The main point is that evidence of memorial processing appears very early in a child's life. This underscores the importance of memory to human functioning, and especially to learning, which is the chief task confronting young children.

Does Early Memory Have a Social Bias?

Of all the things we experience in the world, why do we remember some things better than others? In order to remember things, we need to pay attention to them. As we saw in the previous chapter, attention is influenced by social experiences, especially those of early childhood. Attention involves determining what among all the incoming stimuli is important or worth processing in detail. For young children, much of this attentional sorting is directed and supported by more experienced partners, especially parents. So, too, there is a social character to memory, or a *social bias,* and this bias is evident early in life.

Recognition memory in infancy appears enhanced for perceptual experiences that coincide with the type of input that is social in nature. Even in the first few months of life, infants prefer looking at faces to looking at other objects. This preference is not a consequence of babies liking faces per se, at least not initially. Rather, faces have certain perceptual properties that attract babies' attention, including symmetry, a certain arrangement of main features, and areas of high tonal or color contrast. Dannemiller and Stephens (1988) showed that infants younger than 12 weeks of age prefer visual stimuli that have these properties whether or not they depict human faces. However, by 12 weeks of age, infants appear to identify faces as faces and prefer them over other stimuli, even those with similar perceptual properties.

At about this same age, infants demonstrate a preference for human motion over other forms of movement (Bertenthal, 1993). This preference was studied by showing infants two different light displays, one that looked like a human figure walking and the other that was a random collection of lights. Other senses also show a distinct early bias toward social stimuli—for example, infants have the ability to distinguish the types of audio input that humans produce, like speech sounds (Eimas, Siqueland, Juscyk, & Vigorito, 1971) and tones (Fernald, 1991). Whether infants have better memory for human movement or sounds is not known from these data. However, given selective attention to such stimuli, and therefore increased opportunity to learn and remember this information, this is a reasonable hypothesis.

A bias toward social information clearly facilitates early social and emotional development. For this reason, this is where much of the research on this topic centers. However, this bias also assists early memory development in a very important way. Infants know little about the world when they are born. Thus, a fundamental task of development, especially early in life, is acquiring knowledge about the context in which the child lives (Nelson, 1996). Infants are born with tremendous equipment that sets the stage for psychological development in the early years. In particular, the sensory and motor systems link the infant with the surrounding world. It is good that these systems are so competent at the beginning because the newborn is immediately bombarded by a vast amount and range of incoming information. Learning and development can only proceed if this incoming information is organized and processed in some way. But how is a baby to know what to process and how to organize this input?

Like adults, infants cannot process all incoming information. Selection and sorting is necessary. Some of this selection and sorting appears to be driven by internal processes, such as the types of preferences described above. These preferences may be instrumental in "bootstrapping" early learning (Gottlieb, 1992). In other words, a bias toward other human beings provides opportunities for the young child to learn and develop cognitive skills under the tutelage of a more experienced partner. The protracted course of human dependency helps ensure this connection. Thus, sorting and selecting and learning all sorts of information about the world are largely informed and expedited by someone "who has already been there," who has more experience along the very lines of experience that the baby needs in order to develop the knowledge and skills important for further development.

Thus, other people, especially those more experienced than the infant—which is just about everyone—help the baby learn about the world. They provide babies and young children with much of their experience, they guide them as they direct their attention, and they assist them in processing information. Therefore, it stands to reason that much of early learning and memory is fueled by social experience. The opportunities and constraints provided by the social world work in tandem with the opportunities and constraints of the biological system to shape both the content and the process of the development of memory.

At this point it is important to stress that this claim, namely, that much of what we know, and therefore remember, is organized and supported by social experience, is a hypothesis. A test of this hypothesis needs to demonstrate several things. First, it needs to show that social experiences can impact memory and its development. Second, if children's memory is found to be influenced by social experience, it must determine whether what children learn about remembering from these experiences is uniquely a consequence of social experience or whether it can be acquired in other ways. At the risk of giving away the punch line, no study answers these questions conclusively. However, the collection of studies on this topic point to a singular conclusion, namely, that social experience is instrumental in the early to middle years of childhood for organizing both the content and the process of remembering. This observation underscores the view of memory as a social construction as well as the idea that knowledge acquisition and maintenance are inherently social processes.

THE SOCIAL CONTEXT OF MEMORY DEVELOPMENT

The social construction of memory is common in parent–child interactions as they discuss the past. According to Snow (1990), parents communicate to children what events are worth learning and remembering. Early on in these interactions, parents provide substantial scaffolding for children's participation. When children are very young, parents ask many questions, and in some instances even provide the answers to these questions that they then ask their children to repeat. According to Wertsch (1978), parents assume a role something like an "auxiliary metamemory" for children. That is, parents handle the executive aspects of remembering while children carry out other aspects of remembering that are within their grasp. With time, children assume more responsibility for these social memory activities. Language development plays a critical role in this process (Nelson, 1996). As children develop communicative competence their participation in and contributions to social remembering change. But language development is not the only important component of this process. Changes in children's social and representational skills, as well as changes in children's understanding of self, are also important.

The structure of memory interactions and the way in which adults draw children into conversations about the past are important features of this developmental process. During memory talk, the adult, usually a parent, essentially appropriates or co-opts the child into what Middleton (1997) calls *conversational remembering.* To illustrate, Middleton reports the conversation between a mother and her 4-year-old son as they talked about a family photo. The child, Paul, said very little. However, his mother constantly positioned him as the next speaker. In this way, she evoked the child's memory of the event along with his memory of his emotional state at the time of the event.

> MOTHER: Oh, look, there's when we went to the riding stables, wasn't it?
>
> PAUL: Yeah, er . . . er
>
> MOTHER: You was trying to reach up and stroke that horse.
>
> PAUL: Where? (*Laughs.*)
>
> MOTHER: Would you like to do that again?
>
> PAUL: Yeh.
>
> MOTHER: You don't look very happy though.
>
> PAUL: Because I thought I was going to fall off. (p. 76)

Mother's interest and guidance brought the child's memory forward. They also organized the child's memory and underscored its emotional significance. As this example suggests, children learn about the past and about remembering by participating in social recollections that are orchestrated by an adult in such as way that they tap into the child's region of sensitivity for learning about memory, that is, the child's zone of proximal development. This is consistent with Vygotsky's (1986) view of the development of memory as an emergent social process.

For Vygotsky, social interaction provides human learning and memory with both a "social nature and a process by which children grow into the intellectual life of those around them" (1978, p. 88). Included in this intellectual life are both what the child remembers and the strategies and techniques used to mediate and support memorial processing. These strategies are conveyed to children through opportunities for them to participate in memory activities with other more experienced persons. Learning about and using these memory strategies or mediational means are as much a part of memory development as children's internal memory activities. These mediational means, conveyed through social experience, provide several types of instrumental support for children in this important area of intellectual growth. This raises the question of what functions shared remembering serves.

The Functions of Shared Remembering

The act of sharing memories has many potential benefits for the development of children's memory (see Table 5.1). These include learning how to remember and to share memories with others, shaping the child's self-concept, informing the child about his or her social and cultural history as well as the values of his or her family and community, and promoting social solidarity.

Learning about the Memory Process

One important function of shared remembering is to provide children with opportunities to learn about memory strategies by participating in interactions in which these memory strategies are used. These opportunities can help children develop strategies that they can then use later when they remember the information on their own (Rogoff & Mistry, 1985). For example, in one study (described in more detail below), children who received the most guidance from their mothers in learning how to handle a memory task, especially regarding the organization of the items to be remembered, and had the most opportunities to participate during the interaction in this strategy, performed better on a later recall test that relied on this memorial strategy for success (Rogoff & Gauvain, 1986).

Sharing Memories with Others

The development of one particular type of strategy for remembering that is very useful for recalling everyday events, the narrative form, is aided by social remembering. A *narrative* is a structure for remembering and communicating memories. It contains a unique sequence of

TABLE 5.1. Functions of Shared Remembering in Children's Memory Development

- Children learn about memory processes, for example, strategies.
- Children learn ways of remembering and communicating memories with others, for example, narrative structure.
- Children learn about themselves, which contributes to the development of the self-concept.
- Children learn about their own social and cultural history.
- Children learn values important to the family and the community, that is, what is worth remembering.
- Promotes social solidarity.

events that involve human beings as characters (Bruner, 1986). It can be about a real or an imaginary event and it includes information about the intentionality of the actors, as well as information about the cause and evaluation of the event. The narrative form is often used in every-day conversations about the past, as well as for storing and retrieving information. Narratives appear early and frequently in children's conversations about the past with their parents and other adults. Interestingly, the amount of information contained in the narratives that young children produce can exceed what children of this same age can remember without this memorial structure. Nelson (1996) reports that 23-month-old Emily could recall in correct temporal sequence six different actions from a specific event, such as being awakened at the baby-sitter's house and taken home. This feat would have exceeded memory capacity at this age if a mnemonic technique, such as a narrative structure, had not been used to organize the child's memory.

Development of the Self-Concept

Memory talk may help develop a child's self-concept (Howe, Courage, & Peterson, 1994). In recalling the past, children can characterize what they remember and how they remember their experiences. They can also discover what others find interesting or important in their own history. For example, Engel (1995) describes a 5-year-old boy's description to his mother of a just-completed run with his cousin to the end of the block and back: "We ran down to the end of the road. And I got there first. And then we turned around, and we got here in 30 seconds" (p. 186). The content of this memory, as reported to the mother, will shape what the child remembers about his participation in the event—in this instance, his great success.

Social and Cultural History

Memory talk also informs children about their own social and cultural history. This helps connect children and their lives to other people and to the larger society (Miller & Sperry, 1988). Elder's (1999) research, which examined the impact of the Great Depression and economic hardship on child development, provides a fine example. His data show how the memories of adults who experienced the Depression as children contained both the objective deprivations that they experienced, such as parental unemployment and family dependence on public assistance, and the way that parents talked to their children about family difficulties during this period. Elder also found a positive relation between the frequency that parents discussed these types of experiences during the Depression and the socialization of certain values in the children. These values, maintained well into adulthood, included increased appreciation of social issues, especially in relation to contemporary opportunities and economic security. In other words, different approaches to the past, recorded in family memories, led to different developmental outcomes for children. This is consistent with Reiss's (1981) claim that families remember their own history as a result of how and what they communicate about this past to each other and to the outside world.

Knowledge and Values of the Community

Memory talk also teaches children about the knowledge and values that are important to their family and community. That is, children learn what is worth remembering. For example, Heath (1983) recounts an instance in which a parent from a poor southern community corrected her young child's statement of fact, clearly conveying values about truth and communication in this community. In this example, Teegie, aged 24 months, had just returned from his first haircut, and Heath asked him what he did when he was at the barber shop. Teegie responded by saying "I color." His mother immediately corrected him, saying "You color, huh? You ain't color, you cry." Teegie then said, "I cry." By sharing a memory, the child's recollection was opened to examination. And, in so doing, it was evaluated, in this case for truthfulness, a family and community value, and then it was corrected—a lesson Teegie clearly learned.

Promotion of Social Solidarity

Shared reminiscence may also promote social solidarity among family and other group members (Nelson, 1993). However, because memories are socially constructed, they are more than a sum of the individual memories of the group members. Hirst and Manier (1996) asked family members to recall an important family event individually and then participate in a group recall of this same event. They found that the group recall was more detailed than any one of the family member's individual memories, but that the sum total of all the individual recollections included more detail than the group memory. This suggests that the "family story" is different from each individual member's story. Therefore, the memory of the group is not reducible to any single memory or merely to a summation of individual contributions. Rather, memory was affected by the group dynamics, which led to a unique construction of this memory during family recollection. This suggests that the process of social remembering may promote social solidarity, at least in part, because some of the records or memories of an individual's own experiences are encased in the social world. Social interaction can operate to release these memories, and in so doing it connects the participants in a very interesting way to one another—via avenues to their own past.

These are the primary functions that shared remembering serves in memory development. It is evident that, taken as a whole, the process of shared remembering can inform both the content and the process of memory. Social remembering also connects children to the immediate and broader contexts in which their growth occurs. I now turn to a discussion of research that has examined how social experience may influence the development in childhood of two important types of remembering: event memory and strategic memory.

SOCIAL INFLUENCES ON THE DEVELOPMENT
OF EVENT AND STRATEGIC MEMORY

Two types of memory development have been studied in relation to social influences: event memory and strategic memory. Most research on social influences on memory development in the preschool years concentrates on event and autobiographical memory because it is during this time that much in the development of this type of memory occurs. The social transmission of memory strategies is more evident in the early school years when children acquire and show increased use of many types of mnemonic strategies, including rehearsal and organization.

An important precursor of learning about either of these types of memory from social experience is the understanding that other people rely on memory, both their own and memories that are shared during social activity. Bruner (1990) calls this concept *social agency*. This concept includes awareness that human action is organized around intentional states and that others understand and can help a person carry out activities that rely on shared knowledge or memory. In the development of memory in social context, a sense of social agency is critical. But when does this understanding emerge?

Home observations of infants between 7 and 12 months of age suggest that late in infancy children start to exhibit behaviors that suggest some rudimentary understanding of others as social agents (Ashmead & Perlmutter, 1980). Before describing this research, however, I want to stress that what infants do in these interactions is act *as if* they are developing awareness of social agency. What infants actually understand at this point about other people and their knowledge states is unknown. However, it is the case that infant behavior at this time suggests an emerging, though rudimentary, concept of social agency.

To study infant understanding of social agency, Ashmead and Perlmutter (1980) asked 11 parents to keep home diaries for 6 weeks that recorded any behaviors exhibited by their 7-, 9-, or 11-month-old infants that suggested a past experience. Parents were also asked to indicate whether these instances occurred in or out of the original context of the experience. The researchers were interested in several types of memory-related behaviors including memory of perceptual attributes (e.g., noting a minor change in grandmother's appearance), of the functional attributes of objects or people (e.g., remembering the noise a toy makes), or of the location of objects or people (e.g., pointing out where the dog sleeps). The researchers were also interested in social interactions that were initiated by or responded to by the infant that involved memory. Of primary interest for our discussion are these latter two behaviors. An example of an infant-initiated memory is when an 11-month-old handed his empty cup to his caregiver to fill. An example of a 9-month-old responding to a memory-related act by another person occurred when the child's mother said peekaboo and the child held his bib in front of his face.

In total, 239 memory-related observations were coded (an average of 27 per family); 114 (48%) of these were related to the two types of memory behaviors that involved social interaction. The high rate of social memories is worth noting given the types of "nonsocial" memory events, like object and location memory, included in the observations. Activities involving object and location memory are especially important to infants in the latter half of the first year of life when they are beginning to crawl and move around on their own and show great interest in objects and people, especially primary caregivers. The data suggest that social interactions that are memory-related in some way are just as important as other types of memories, such as those involving space and object exploration, that emerge during this time.

Another interesting finding from this research is that memory-related behaviors initiated by the infants increased over the ages studied, especially between 7 and 9 months. Table 5.2 contains the frequency for the different age groups of these two types of social memories. Most of these memories (close to two-thirds) involved the infant anticipating either a positive or an aversive interaction with another person. Ashmead and Perlmutter provided the following diary entry from the mother of a 7-month-old as an example.

"John has his first cold and has had to have his nose wiped repeatedly, which he dislikes. After his meal, I usually use a washcloth to wash his

TABLE 5.2. Average Number of Infant Memory-Related Behaviors Reported by Parents over a 6-Week Period by Age of Child

Age of child	Infant memory-related behaviors	
	Infant initiated	Infant responded
7 months	4	32
9 months	19	20
11 months	18	21

Note. Data from Ashmead and Perlmutter (1980).

hands, then his face. As soon as I began to wash his hands, he responded by pulling his hands to his face and turning his face away from me." (p. 13)

Observations such as this suggest that by the time children begin to talk, they are already engaged in interactions with adults that imply some rudimentary sense of social agency and that involve acting on memory in the course of social acts. After the infancy period, these interactions are enriched considerably by the child's emerging linguistic and representational competence. Research has shown that during early childhood the linkage between social interaction and early memory development is evident in children's emerging event and autobiographical memory.

Event and Autobiographical Memory

In 1990, Katherine Nelson commented that most research on children's memory concludes that children under 5 years of age have poor memories. However, according to Nelson, if parents were asked about their young children's memory, most would report that their children have very good memories, especially for experienced events. Personal experiences are important to development. Therefore, it is not surprising that memory for these events appears early in childhood. Why were such memories, until recently, overlooked in research?

The answer tells more about the history of the field than the developmental process itself. In part a lack of appreciation of memory skills in early childhood may have been fueled by a conception of preschool children as cognitively inept. For many years preschool children were seen as possessing only rudimentary intellectual skills. This view influenced the nature of research with this age group (Gelman, 1979). At this time, if preschool children were included in research, they were typically positioned as a comparison group for describing the competencies of early school-age children. The name of Piaget's second stage of mental development, *preoperational*, implies this view by referring to what preschool children cannot do rather than to what they can do. Fortunately, over the last decades this trend has reversed and a large body of research on young children's cognitive development has appeared, including research on the development of event and autobiographical memory during this period.

Event memory concerns things that happen in everyday life. It involves explicit awareness that something is being remembered. Because event memories are often complex in the number of actions they include, the sequencing of these actions, and their temporal qualities, the memory of events is greatly aided by the use of a narrative structure. As noted above, a narrative is a specialized form of organizational strategy. It follows a temporal sequence and includes information about the intentions and personal involvement of the actors in the story. It also contains routinized knowledge, like scripts, as a general frame of reference. Script knowledge can be used to "jump-start" a memory if it wanes or gets off track somewhere along the way. For example, a child may not remember what came next when the family went out to dinner, so a conversational partner may probe the child's memory by asking if certain scripted events, like whether menus were brought to the table or the family had a salad before the main course, occurred.

What early skills may contribute to the development of event memories that are based on a narrative structure? One important contribution to the child's developing ability to participate in and generate narratives is the understanding of temporal and causal relations. Research by Bauer and Mandler (1990) shows that children as young as 16 months of age are sensitive to the temporal and causal order of events. They demonstrated this by showing children one of two novel events. One event, the Frog Jump, involved three different objects: a wooden board, a wedge-shaped block, and a toy frog. An experimenter presented these materials to some of the infants and showed them how to lean the board against the block to make a teeter-totter. The experimenter then placed the frog on the board, hit it, and caused the frog "to jump." Other infants in this study were shown another novel event, one that lacked a causal organization. For example, some children were asked to make a picture and were given a small chalkboard, a piece of chalk, a sticker, and an easel. The experimenter showed the child how to attach the sticker to the chalkboard, lean the chalkboard against the easel, and scribble on the chalkboard. When the children were later asked to recall the novel events, they had better memory for events that contained temporal and causal relations among elements. This suggests that as early as 16 months of age children are better at remembering events that have an inherent temporal structure, a tendency ideally suited to event and autobiographical memory. Thus, by the toddler period, children are capable of understanding the basic narrative form. Do children of this age have opportunity to develop event memories in the social setting that encompasses most of their daily experience, namely, the family?

Researchers estimate that during family interaction discussion of past events occur as often as five to seven times an hour (Fivush, Haden, & Reese, 1996). Parents talk directly to children about the past. Parents also talk to each other about the past in their children's presence, and children talk about the past to their parents and other adults. Early in the child's life shared memories are mostly one-sided, with the parent taking on much of the responsibility for reminiscing. But by the age of 3, children's contributions to shared remembering increase. Also, around this time memories begin to endure rather well. Children as young as 3 years of age can remember specific event information over a fairly long time period (Fivush & Hamond, 1989; Hamond & Fivush, 1991), as the following example indicates. Three-year-old Benjamin tells his grandmother about his family's move across the country on a train, which occurred when he was 2½:

BEN: We rode on the train for 3 whole days, and, and I slept with my mommy on the high bed.

GRANDMOTHER: Where was Graeme [Ben's baby brother]?

BEN: Graeme slept on the floor in a basket and the bathroom was next to him.

This recollection is similar to the type observed by Hamond and Fivush (1991) when they interviewed preschoolers 6 to 18 months following a visit to Disneyworld. The children went to the theme park when they were either 3 or 4 years of age. Even though the older children recalled more details, all the children recalled a substantial amount of information about the trip, even with a gap of 18 months between the experience and the report.

According to Hudson (1990), conversations between parents and children contribute in significant ways to the development of autobiographical memory. To investigate this, Hudson conducted a 7-month case study of conversations between her and her daughter Rachel when Rachel was between 21 and 28 months of age. When Rachel was 21 months old, these conversations consisted mostly of yes and no questions about the past, with the questions initiated by her mother. For example:

MOTHER: And did you have ice cream?

RACHEL: Yes. Ice cream. (p. 180)

When Rachel was 24 months old, she began contributing more information to these conversations, though they were still primarily initiated by her mother, as in the following example:

MOTHER: Did you like the apartment at the beach?

RACHEL: Yeah. And I have fun in the water. (p. 180)

Here Rachel added some of her own memories to the conversation. By the time she was 27 months old, Rachel was initiating more of these conversations, as in the following exchange:

RACHEL: Do you remember the waves, Mommy?

MOTHER: Do I remember the waves? What about the waves?

RACHEL: I go in the waves and I build a sandcastle. And do you remember we swimmed? I swimmed in the waves and we did it again. Did we play again? (p. 181)

Over this 7-month period, Rachel learned quite a bit about how to remember from these conversations. In particular, she learned how to participate in them and, toward the end of the period, how to initiate talk about the past.

These same age-related patterns were reflected in a study that Hudson (1990) conducted with a group of 10 mothers and children over a 4-week period when the children were between 24 and 30 months of age. Hudson found that early in the observational period, the children, like Rachel, had limited ability to talk about past events. They were mainly dependent on their mothers to cue these memories. However, once their memories were activated and they had more experience in these conversations, the children became active participants, and what's more, their contributions did not simply repeat what their mothers had said but sometimes included new information about the event. This suggests that in the second year of life children are beginning to recollect past experiences. However, these memorial activities occur in conversations that are heavily scaffolded by adults and they are organized around a narrative structure.

Observations such as these are consistent with other research that shows that children are participating in conversations that include event memories in the early years of childhood. This begs the question of whether these experiences help children develop, organize, and maintain these memories. One answer to this is that these conversations do help children retain memory for these particular events. For example, Hamond and Fivush (1991) showed that children who talked more about events with their parents had better memory for the event. Elder's (1999) research on adult memories of the Great Depression shows a similar pattern. The other, related, question is whether these experiences influence the development of children's event memory more generally.

Research by Ratner (1980, 1984) addresses this question. This research involved children between the ages of 24 and 42 months. Ratner was interested in the links between memory demands made by mothers when they talked with their children about past events and the children's later memory performance on other types of memory tasks. In order to examine this topic, she conducted four home observations over a 2-week period and tape-recorded the conversations of mothers and children as they went about their daily routines. Following the observational period, the children participated in a laboratory memory task that involved remembering the rooms and furnishings in a dollhouse. The home observations revealed that mothers frequently talk about past events to children in this age range. Much of this talk occurs in question form, a technique designed to engage the conversational partner in the discussion. About one-quarter of the mothers' total speech to children was formulated as questions, and two-thirds of these questions were about past events. In most cases, these questions were about events that had just occurred. However, 14% of these types of questions referred to events farther in the past.

How did children's experience with memory conversations at home relate to their memory performance in the lab? For the 2-year-olds, there was no relation. However, for the 3-year-olds, there was a positive relation between the frequency with which mothers posed event questions at home and children's memory in the lab. This relation was qualified in that only questions about remote, not immediate, past events were related to better memory performance in the lab. For Ratner, this relation is not surprising in that discussing remote events and remembering the location of rooms and furnishings in a dollhouse both rely on the same memorial process, namely, retrieval from long-term storage. Interestingly, children whose mothers asked many questions about recent events performed poorly on the lab memory task. This suggests that it is not the asking of questions per se that is the important link between social and individual memory performance. Rather, it is asking questions about past events that requires children to retrieve information not recently experienced that is important.

These results suggest that the memory processes of children as young as 3 years of age can benefit from conversations with adults.

However, it is important to note, as Ratner does, that the direction of influence is unknown. Children's own memory abilities may have influenced the memory demands that mothers made on them at home, as well as the children's memory performance in the lab. In other words, mothers may talk more to young children about the past if the mothers believe or have evidence that their children have good memories of such events.

In addition to the contributions of children's individual memory abilities to this process, research shows that the narrative form itself may benefit the development of children's event memory. Tessler and Nelson (1994) audiotaped the conversations of 10 mothers and their 3- to 3½-year-old children when they visited a museum. Mothers were randomly assigned to one of two conditions: half the mothers were asked to interact normally with their children, the remainder were asked to respond only to their children's questions. One week later the children were interviewed by an experimenter and asked about their museum visit. The interview included free recall followed by specific questions about the visit. Analysis of the children's memory during the interview showed that none of the children recalled anything they saw in the museum but did not talk about with their mother. Furthermore, children only remembered objects that both the mother and the child discussed. Children did not remember what the mother talked about on her own (without engaging the child) or what the child commented on alone (without a response from mother).

This type of evidence suggests that children's event memory develops, in large part, in social context and through social interactions of particular sorts. It leads directly to the question Would children's event memories be formulated or retained without parental or adult assistance? Undoubtedly they would be, at least to some degree. No one believes that young children's memory for events is entirely dependent on conversations with adults, although this is an empirical (though not readily testable) question. However, as with adults, the less children are reminded of or rehearse their memories by reflecting on them or relating them to others, the less likely it is that they will be remembered. Also, as with adults, the less organized memories are, the less likely they are to be remembered.

The important distinction in comparing the process of organizing and maintaining memories that is experienced by young children relative to adults is the fact that children often need assistance in retrieving and organizing these memories. Research suggests that adults are willing, able, and frequent participants in guiding children through this process. Adults help children develop event memory skills by talking to them about the past, encouraging children to add their own knowledge to these conversations, and providing children with practice using an organizational scheme for these memories—the narrative form—that facilitates the development and organization of remembering. In other words, parents help children remember events in a way that makes them easier for the child to remember as well as more amenable to sharing with others.

The fact that these conversations typically tie these memories to something of personal or social significance to the child helps children acquire knowledge about themselves, other people, and the world they live in. Furthermore, this type of personal "storytelling," or shared reminiscence, is not unique to particular families or cultures. It is a practice that is culturally widespread and valued (Miller & Moore, 1989). This suggests that social remembering between children and adults serves broader cultural goals, along the very lines suggested by Shotter (1990). That is, by sharing memories and learning to share memories with others, children become connected to the knowledge of their community as well as to the ways of organizing, maintaining, and communicating this knowledge that are valued in their community, both in local familial terms and in the larger cultural context.

Some research supports the view that the early conversations that parents and children have about past events reflect cultural values. Mullen and Yi (1995) observed 16 mother–child dyads in which the children were between 37 and 44 months of age. Half of the dyads were Korean and half were European American. Home recordings were made of mother–child conversations about the past. Results indicate a higher rate of conversations about the past among European American dyads than among Korean dyads. In fact, conversations about the past occurred about three times more frequently in the European American dyads than in the Korean dyads. More interesting than the rate of these conversations was their focus. European American mothers made more references to the thoughts and feelings of the children in their memory talk than Korean mothers did. In contrast, Korean mothers included more references to social norms in their memory talk with their children. These patterns are consistent with socialization goals and values in these communities. They suggest that during mother–child conversations about the past, children learn not only how to organize memories for communication, they also learn what aspects of the past are important to talk about, emphasize, and remember.

Is the Second to Third Year a Growth Point for Event Memory?

The research described above suggests that the period between 2 and 3 years of age may be particularly important for the development of event

and autobiographical memory. This period features a unique convergence of several important factors that contribute to this developmental
process. In particular, children's emerging social and representational
skills, along with their increasing linguistic competence, set the stage for
the development of memory in social context. Furthermore, at this same
time children's social life is expanding, especially the types of social interactions and conversations that children have with adults. Much of this
talk involves a give-and-take of information by the participants, and these
conversations often include discussion about the past.

Competence at language, which is changing at a rapid pace at this
very point in development, plays an especially important role in that it
allows for changes in the nature and extent of children's participation
in conversations about the past. Thus, it is not surprising that some of
the same patterns observed in language development during this period are evident in children's early conversations about the past. For example, girls engage in more memory conversations with parents than
boys do (Reese & Fivush, 1993). In terms of representational skills, children's understanding of temporality and causality, along with their developing understanding of routines and events, such as script knowledge (Nelson & Gruendel, 1981), are increasing. These, too, contribute
to event memory and its development, as demonstrated in research by
Welch-Ross (1997). Preschoolers with higher levels of representational
understanding about events (i.e., children who had better understanding of the event from different perspectives, including that of the child
him- or herself, the conversational partner, and what the child was like
in the past when the event occurred) were more active participants in
conversations about the past than children with lower representational
levels of events. These emerging and converging skills make important
contributions to conversations about the past that young children have
with more experienced partners.

Research indicates that not all conversations about the past between
adults and children have the same outcome. Parents have different styles
of talking to their children about the past. Studies have examined how
these styles relate to children's memory. This research is important in
that it investigates social experience not as a global and necessarily beneficial aspect of development, but as a mechanism of cognitive development that can be studied in terms of its properties and how these properties may relate to specific developmental outcomes.

Parental Styles of Talking about the Past

In her research on the development of the narrative form in early
childhood, Engel (1986) found that mothers vary in the amount and

type of memory talk in which they engage with their young children. Some parents talk to their preschool children quite a bit about the past, others much less so. Engel also identified two different styles of reminiscing, or talking about the past, among mothers. Mothers with a *pragmatic style* (which in some of the research below is referred to as a "repetitive style") concentrate on practical matters and facts, as in the following example:

MOTHER: Who came to the birthday party?

CHILD: Bobby and Joe.

MOTHER: Did you eat cake?

CHILD: Yeah.

MOTHER: Was it fun?

CHILD: Yeah.

MOTHER: That's good.

Mothers with an *elaborative style* tend to communicate with their children about the past as more of a story. Moreover, the mother's talk tends to encourage the child's participation in these stories, as in the following example:

MOTHER: What did you do at the birthday party?

CHILD: We found hidden treasure.

MOTHER: You did? Were these treasures nice?

CHILD: Yeah, they were chocolate.

MOTHER: Were the treasures hard to find?

CHILD: They were all over . . . in corners and under pillows. I found two, Bobby got two too.

Mothers who use an elaborative style essentially create, and engage their children in, a narrative about the event.

Both these styles have been identified in several studies examining mother–child conversations about the past (Haden, 1998; Hudson, 1990; Reese, Haden, & Fivush, 1993). In one study these styles were shown to be used by both mothers and fathers when they talk with their young children about the past. Interestingly, in this research, parents of daughters tended to use an elaborative style more than parents of sons (Reese & Fivush, 1993), which is consistent with the finding that girls engage in more memory conversations with parents than boys do. These gender-related conversational patterns appear reciprocal or mutual in form.

In all of the research on parental style of reminiscence the same pattern has been observed. These styles encourage different types of memory talk from children. When a parent uses an elaborative style of reminiscing, children take longer conversational turns and their contributions include more memory elaborations, repetitions, and evaluations (either confirming or negating the parent's prior utterance) than when a parent uses a pragmatic or repetitive style. In addition, a repetitive style is associated with less responding by the child during memory-related conversations (see Table 5.3). These two styles also relate differently to the child's later individual memory performance. Children of parents who use an elaborative style remember more on later individual memory tests than children of parents who use a pragmatic or repetitive style, and these patterns are independent of the children's linguistic ability (Haden, 1998). This suggests that different ways of interacting with young children about past events have different consequences for how children engage in these interactions and what children may learn about memory from these exchanges.

The discussion so far has concentrated on the cognitive developmental aspects of social remembering. It stresses that the child's increasing memorial, linguistic, and representational competence set the stage for learning about memory in social context. Furthermore, it suggests that the consequences of these experiences for child development are cognitive in nature as children learn about the content and process of remembering. There are other important contributions to this process. These include changes in the child's social skills that allow these social interactions to occur. Unfortunately, these changes have not been the focus of much research. In addition, emotional development is part of this process. Much of what children discuss with parents in

TABLE 5.3. Correlations between Parental Reminiscence Styles and Child Participation in Parent–Child Memory Conversations

Child behavior	Parental style	
	Elaborative	Repetitive
Length of utterance	.90**	.15
Memory elaborations	.75**	.13
Repetitions	.82**	.14
Evaluations	.56**	.05
Off-topic comments	.14	.16
No response	.27	.38*

Note. From Reese and Fivush (1993). Copyright 1993 by the American Psychological Association. Adapted by permission.

these conversations are topics of personal importance to the child. Moreover, the participants themselves are important to each other. Again, little is known about the emotional aspects of these conversations and how these may relate to the development of memory. One area of socioemotional development has been explored in relation to the emergence of autobiographical memory: the development of the self system. This is included in my discussion of parental styles of reminiscing because one study on this topic did a particularly good job of distinguishing the contributions of parental styles of reminiscing and children's emerging self-awareness to the development of event memory in young children.

According to Howe and Courage (1993), children's developing understanding of the self, which appears in the second year of life, is a critical facet of the emergence of autobiographical memory. This view was challenged by Harley and Reese (1999). They conceded that the development of the self is one part of the development of autobiographical memory, but argued that parental contributions and the child's linguistic ability are also critical. To investigate this topic, Harley and Reese examined the relation between maternal reminiscence style and children's self-knowledge, verbal skill, and autobiographical memory. This short-term longitudinal study involved mothers and their children, who were observed at 19, 25, and 32 months of age. All the data were collected in home visits. At the initial visit, the children's verbal skill and the mothers' style of reminiscing were assessed. Maternal reminiscence style was rated as either low or high on elaborative memory talk. Children's self-concept was assessed using a standard mirror identification task (Lewis & Brooks-Gunn, 1979). Half of the children in the study identified themselves in the mirror and half did not; these two groups were identified as early and late, respectively, in the development of the self system. At the second and third visits, children discussed memory events with the experimenter. The children's utterances were classified as either memory elaborations, that is, as providing new information about a remembered event, or memory repetitions, that is, as restating information previously told to them by another.

Results indicate that independent of the child's verbal skill, both maternal style of reminiscing and children's self-awareness are important predictors of children's event memory. However, these two factors predicted children's memory in different contexts. Replicating earlier research, maternal reminiscing style was the best predictor of children's memory elaborations when the children talked with their mothers about a shared memory. However, child self-recognition was the best predictor of the child's independent elaborations of event memory when talking with the experimenter. These findings suggest that developmental processes other than the child's linguistic competence and the nature of parent–child conversations about the past, such as the development of the self system, may play important roles in the development of event memory in young children.

In sum, research suggests that adults, especially parents, provide guidance for young children during their conversations about the past that contributes to the development of event and autobiographical memory. Conversations about the past, and the narrative structure they assume, compose a substantial portion of young children's experience with adults, especially parents, during the early years of childhood. The narrative form is useful for organizing event knowledge in children's memory as well as for helping them communicate with others about the past. Individual variation in both the content and style of parent–child conversations about the past exists, and these have different consequences for the types of memory experiences children have and the opportunities children have to develop memory skills in social context. In addition to the narrative form, adults communicate much information to children in these conversations about the past, including the importance of recollecting events with others. Such shared memory experiences carry much import in young children's lives. They contribute to the development of the self, and thereby help create what Nelson (1996) calls the *historical self*. They also contribute to the development of the *cultural self* in that these shared memory experiences direct both the content and the process of remembering along lines valued by the community in which development occurs.

We now turn to research on another aspect of memory development that also bears the stamp of social influences: the development of strategic memory.

Strategic Memory

Vygotsky (1978) discussed two basic types of memory. *Natural memory* involves the immediate processing of incoming stimuli. It is not mediated by signs, symbols, or social experience. He thought of this as very similar to perceptual processing and expected little variation across cultures. The other type of memory, which Vygotsky considered a higher level mental function, is *mediated memory*. This involves remembering that extends beyond the limitations of basic psychological functions and relies on culturally elaborated ways, or strategies, for organizing and supporting memory development and use. *Strategies* are deliberate behaviors used to enhance memory performance (Naus & Ornstein, 1983).

Cultures vary in the extent to which they support and encourage children's participation in particular memory strategies (Mistry, 1997). In Western societies, children, especially those of school age, are often required to use strategies to remember information. This is because, in simplified terms, formal schooling involves the processing of large amounts of information and this information is typically presented in a form that is difficult to remember without the use of overt and explicit strategies. (See Goody, 1977, for discussion of the cognitive demands and consequences associated with remembering large amounts of information that appear in abstract and decontextualized form.) Strategies such as rehearsal, organization, and elaboration are especially useful for this purpose. These strategies are less common among children and adults in non-Western cultures, who are more skilled than Westerners at using spatial and narrative strategies to encode and recall information. Thus, cultural practices influence the types of memorial strategies that children develop.

These strategies are communicated to children, or mediated by, social experience. For example, Australian Aborigine children have to learn important information about their desert environment, such as the location of water holes. Writer Bruce Chatwin (1987) searched for the origin and meaning of the Australian Aboriginal Songline, which is a traditional record of important memories and ideas, including important locations. An expert informant in the region explained the following to him: "Each totemic ancestor was thought to have scattered a trail of words and musical notes along the line of his footprints . . . these Dreaming-tracks lay over the land as 'ways' of communication between the most far-flung tribes. A song was both a map and a direction-finder" (p. 13). Chatwin went on to discover that Aboriginal mothers teach young children about Songlines. Mothers draw sketches in the sand and use these to illustrate the wanderings of the Dreamtime heroes. In this way Aboriginal children learn to "orient themselves to the land, its mythology and resources" (p. 22). In other words, this is a way of teaching children to remember important information in this community.

The social contributions to strategic memory have been studied by developmental psychologists with children ranging in age from toddlerhood to late childhood. This research typically involves observations of the interactions of adults—often parents—and children. Sometimes this research includes individual memory tests for the children before and after the interaction to examine how the social experience contributes to the development of children's memory skills. Studies examining peer influences on the development of memory strategies are rare, at least in the early to middle years of childhood. (Incidentally, this is a burgeoning area of research among those who study adult memory [Weldon & Bellinger, 1997], and would certainly be interesting to explore with adolescents.) However, some research does include comparisons of adult–child and peer collaboration on tasks involving memory.

Perez-Granados and Callanan (1997) studied the interactions of preschool peers and Ellis and Rogoff (1982) studied the interactions of children in middle childhood. Both studies compared peer interaction to adult–child interaction on the same tasks. These studies found a similar pattern, namely, that adults provide more opportunity than peers for children to participate in and learn memory strategies during joint cognitive activity. This may be due to the fact that peers talk less to each other than adults and children do when they work together. Because verbal exchange is important, especially in Western communities, for transmitting strategy information, this may account for much of the observed difference. However, research suggests that in some circumstances children will teach memory strategies to other children. Best and Ornstein (1986) asked third- and sixth-grade children to teach first graders how to remember the items in a picture. Older children who were previously taught a useful memory strategy for this task, namely, an organization of the items in the picture, were more likely to convey this strategy information to the first graders than older children who had not been taught this strategy information. This suggests that, at least in certain circumstances, school-age children are able to communicate memory strategies effectively to younger children. However, because of the limited amount of research on peer influences on the development of memory strategies, the remainder of my discussion focuses on adult influences on this development.

Children under 5 years of age are in the beginning stages of strategy acquisition. Some interesting and important strategies are formulated during the preschool years, including naming, pointing, and selective attention. For example, DeLoache, Cassidy, and Brown (1985) observed 18- to 24-month-olds as they tried to remember the location of a Big Bird doll they had seen hidden just a few minutes earlier in their homes. The children used a number of strategies to remember the location, including staring at the hiding place, pointing at it, and naming the hidden object. These strategies all helped keep the object and its location "in the child's mind" during the waiting period, as evidenced by the children's later performance. Children who used these strategies were more successful at retrieving the toy when the waiting period was up.

Few studies have examined social influences on the development of memory strategies in the preschool years. There is some suggestion that late in this period when children are beginning to use rudimentary forms of strategies that aid memory, like selective attention, social experience may be a contributing factor in the development of these skills. Preschoolers are more likely to use strategies like selective attention when adults help them carry out tasks that are cognitively demanding than when children of this age do these tasks on their own (Miller, Woody-Ramsey, & Aloise, 1991). Guidance from an adult apparently mediates the children's capacity limitations, and thereby provides children with the opportunity to use strategies of which they are knowledgeable but are too overwhelmed because of task demands to use—what Miller (1990) refers to as a *utilization deficiency*. In addition to a partner relieving the child of some of the task activities, social experience may also encourage the use of memory strategies among preschoolers by reminding the child to use the strategies. Children as young as 3½ to 4½ years of age will use memory strategies, like pointing and manipulating the to-be-remembered items, when they are instructed to do so by an adult during a memory task (Fletcher & Bray, 1996). Together, these findings suggest that strategic memory development in preschoolers may benefit in several ways from the guidance provided by more experienced partners. Since these children are just at the cusp of developing many of the more complex memory strategies evident among school-age children, guidance from adults may be essential during the preschool period in order for children to have the opportunity to learn and practice these strategies.

Between the ages of 5 and 10 years, children acquire a wide range of more complex memory strategies (Siegler, 1998). These include rehearsal, organization, and elaboration. With increasing age over this period of development, children become more skilled in the use of each of these strategies. They are able to use them in a broader range of circumstances, and to use them more effectively and more efficiently. A number of factors contribute to these age-related changes, including maturational contributions in speed of processing and memory capacity. Increases in content knowledge, the emergence of metamemory, and increased self-regulation also occur over these years (Schneider & Bjorkland, 1998); these contribute as well.

Given the sociocultural nature of strategic memory (Vygotsky, 1978), it is not surprising that research has shown that certain cultural practices, like schooling (Rogoff, 1981) and familiar routines for organizing knowledge (Kearins, 1981; Rogoff & Waddell, 1982), also influence the development and use of memory strategies during these years. Social interaction can also facilitate children's use of memory strategies in middle childhood. For instance, in one study, mothers and their 6- to 8-year-old children worked on one of two versions of a memory task (Ellis & Rogoff, 1982). Each task involved identifying and sorting 18 items that could be grouped into six categories. In the home version, the items were groceries that needed to be placed on particular shelves. In the school version, the items were photographs of common household objects that needed to be placed in six specified compartments in a box. During the interaction, the mother taught the child the locations of the items using a cue sheet given to her by the experimenter. This sheet indicated the item placements but did not provide any rationale for the groupings. Following the interaction, the child individually sorted eight of the original items and 12 new items aligned with the categories. Therefore, children had to remember the item locations, the item categories, and their locations to be successful at this task.

In general, mothers provided their children with much mnemonic information about the organization or grouping of the items. Mothers often referred to familiar contexts to help children organize their learning and memory of the items (Rogoff & Gardner, 1984). For example, one mother said to her child, "See, that's the way we do it at home, isn't it? . . . We have all the baking supplies and stuff in one area, don't we?" Other mnemonic aids were also provided by mothers, including elaboration, as in the following example in which a mother's verbal elaboration is supported by her nonverbal behaviors:

MOTHER: What's that?

CHILD: It's a bucket, and it helps you carry things and . . . (*fidgeting*).

MOTHER: Yeah, and it helps you clean (*looking at child*).

CHILD: (*Nods.*)

MOTHER: Okay, what else? Do you see something else that helps you clean? (*Adjusts broom in the cleaning box.*)

CHILD: (*Watches his mother's hand on bucket, then points to bucket, then to broom.*)

MOTHER: The broom, so it should be put in here. (*Holds bucket in cleaning box.*)

CHILD: (*taking bucket from mother's hand and placing it in correct box*) Yeah. (Rogoff & Gardner, 1984, p. 111)

Did maternal guidance about memory strategies facilitate children's use of these strategies in their later individual memory performance? To examine this issue, Rogoff and Gauvain (1986) divided the children into three groups based on their posttest scores: low, intermediate, and high scorers. Table 5.4 shows these groups in relation to the type and extent of cognitive assistance they received from mothers. The investigators found that children who did the best on the posttest (high scorers) received the most guidance from their mothers in terms of the correct organization of the items. These children were provided with category labels for the items, they participated in the task activities at a higher level (specifically, they were involved in making decisions about the categories to which the items belonged), and they were involved in some type of test preparation that involved rehearsing the items and categories. Fifty percent of the children with low scores on the posttest had not been taught the correct organization of the items by their mothers, nor were they involved in any test preparation. Furthermore, none of the children with low scores participated in item placement decisions during the interaction. Thus, these children had less assistance and participation during the interaction to help them learn about strategies for remembering the items. Children with intermediate scores on the posttest had moderate levels of exposure to the correct organization of the items during mother–child interaction, in some cases they were involved in determining the categories of the items, and in most cases they had preparation for the test. These data indicate that adult assistance in the use of an organizational strategy to aid memory was related to children's later performance on an independent memory task with a related group of items. The data also show that without such experience, 6- to 8-year-olds did not spontaneously generate organizational schemes that helped them on the later individual memory task. Working with the items without strategic assistance or simply watching mother group the items did not help the children remember the items. Thus, both strategic assistance from an adult and active participation by the child were crucial for children to develop memory strategies on this task.

Other research involving children of this same age have findings consistent with these results. Kurtz, Schneider, Carr, Borkowski, and Rellinger (1990) observed that second- and third-grade children in Germany use certain memory strategies, in particular sorting and clustering, more than children in the United States. However, after U.S. children were trained to use these strategies, no differences emerged. Questionnaire responses obtained from the parents and teachers of the children indicated that the initial differences may have been due to differences in the instructional strategies that children in these two communities are exposed to at home and at school. This suggests that prior experience with other people, in both formal and informal learning settings, can influence children's acquisition and use of memory strategies during the years of middle childhood when much in the way of strategy development is occurring.

What is it about social interaction that may lead to increased strategic memory in children? Most accounts focus on the exchange of strategic knowledge that occurs either directly, as when an experienced

TABLE 5.4. Proportion of Low, Intermediate, and High Scorers on the Individual Memory Posttest in Relation to Parental Guidance and Child Participation during Parent–Child Interaction

Interaction behavior	Low scorers ($n = 6$)	Intermediate scorers ($n = 15$)	High scorers ($n = 11$)
Mother provided correct organization of items	50%	60%	100%
Moderate to high levels of child participation in item placement decisions	0%	20%	100%
Test preparation at end of interaction	50%	73%	82%

Note. Data from Rogoff and Gauvain (1986).

partner instructs the child in a strategy, or indirectly, as when an experienced partner models a strategy in the child's presence and facilitates the child's participation in this strategy. In both cases the child's current skills serve as a guide to the child's needs. The child's active participation, especially the child's attention to the activity and the strategies used, enables adults to fine-tune their assistance. It also enables children to learn the strategies.

In addition to direct and indirect learning processes, there is also some suggestion that children's memory of social interaction may contribute to individual cognitive change. Foley, Passalacqua, and Ratner (1993) observed the interactions of children and an adult experimenter as they made two different collages (one was identifiable as an animal and one was abstract). The experimenter regulated the interaction to ensure that the partners took turns making the collages. After the interaction, children were interviewed about the activity; in particular, they were asked who was responsible for placing each of the pieces. Because the activity was shared, the researchers hypothesized that the partners would anticipate each other's actions. This, they reasoned, might increase the likelihood that children would confuse who did which action and perhaps lead to misappropriations in the child's memory of the actions of the partner—the "I did it" phenomenon.

The results suggest that this is the case, at least for young children. Four-year-olds, but not 6- and 8-year-old children, were more likely to claim that they placed a piece that the experimenter had actually placed than they were to claim the opposite: that the experimenter placed a piece that the child had actually placed. In a follow-up experiment, the researchers found that the tendency among the 4-year-olds to misappropriate the actions of another only occurred when the adult and child collaborated. If the adult placed the pieces out of the child's view, few misattributions occurred. It is interesting that this pattern appeared for preschoolers only. Later research investigated if this was due to a response tendency by young children to claim responsibility for any actions, regardless of source (Foley & Ratner, 1998). But this apparently is not the case. Preschoolers were more likely to claim "I did it" when a piece was placed by the experimenter, but they did not claim responsibility for pieces that were not placed by either the child or the experimenter (new or distracter pieces).

Why did young children encode and remember shared events in this way? Recall that when preschoolers try to remember they must contend with limitations in both the speed of processing and in memory capacity. Perhaps, as the researchers suggest, recoding the partner's actions as their own may facilitate young children's memory of the task and how to do it. This would allow children to retain important information about how to do the task, but would omit unimportant information (at least "unimportant" in terms of reproducing the actions), like who did what. This results in a simplified memory, one that contains the sequence of the behaviors as a single set of actions done by one person. Such "streamlined" memories may be especially useful for young children for whom remembering both the activity and the participants' actions would be overwhelming. They may prove especially useful on later occasions when the child tries to reproduce these behaviors on his or her own. The fact that the collaboration resulted in a successful performance—that is, the collages were completed—may have also contributed. Whether children would show the same bias in remembering an unsuccessful cognitive activity is not known.

What this research suggests is that, in addition to direct and indirect learning opportunities, other mechanisms of cognitive change tied to social interaction help children learn cognitive skills, like memory strategies, from working with others. This research also suggests that some mechanisms of change may be age-related: they may be more likely to occur, or to benefit children, at certain points in development.

In sum, research suggests that children can learn about memory strategies, like rehearsal and organization, from collaborating with others. Mechanisms of this learning include direct instruction, as adults teach children what these strategies are and how to use them, and less direct approaches, as adults arrange situations in ways that provide children with exposure to and practice with memory strategies. Active participation by the child appears especially important in this learning process.

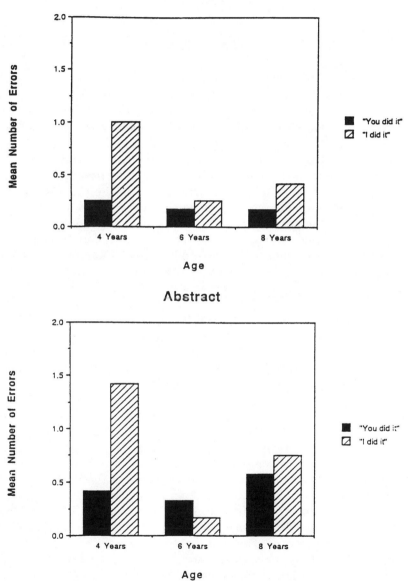

FIGURE 5.2. Mean number of children's misattribution errors following adult–child collaboration making two types of collages by child age. From Foley, Passalacqua, and Ratner (1993). Copyright 1993 by Elsevier Science. Reprinted by permission.

For younger children, a personal misattribution bias may compensate for memory limitations in facilitating such learning in social context.

CONCLUDING THOUGHTS

A recent review of research on memory development identified the factors that result in a good memory (Pressley, Borkowski, & Schneider, 1987). Pressley and colleagues call this the *good information-processing model*. One of its central components is the role that interactional processes play in the acquisition of strategic and metacognitive knowledge. This view is consistent with the research discussed in this chapter in which the development of both the content and the process of memory is described as a socially co-constructed process. The claim is not that social experience is the only way in which children learn memory strategies. Rather, the claim is that it is one, albeit very important, way in which this learning occurs. Through interaction with adults and peers, children learn what things in their own life, their family, and their community are important to remember. They also learn about deliberate techniques that aid remembering, that is, strategies for storing and retrieving memories for later use. Furthermore, the social nature of memory development connects children to their community and culture in ways that provide support for further learning.

This process proceeds in an orderly developmental fashion. Certain maturational skills that facilitate the social co-construction of memory, such as mental representation, linguistic competence, and metacognition, help set the timetable. Other developmentally related skills, like social competence and emotional regulation, also help steer the course. The fact that much of early remembering is done in collaboration with individuals who are of great emotional importance to children, especially parents and siblings, enhances the salience of this entire process. Children are not only learning about the world in which they live, they are learning about it from people who have great meaning to them. Also significant is the fact that much of what children learn about remembering during the early years is rooted in memories of personal experiences. This also makes the process of remembering more salient. It seems clear that the relational and autobiographical nature of these early social remembering experiences arouse the child's motivation in these learning contexts, and thereby facilitates memory development.

The next chapter examines the social process involved in another important area of cognitive development during childhood: problem solving.

Solving and Learning to Solve Problems in Social Context

*I*n 1956, Piaget and Inhelder published a book that described children's ability at tying knots. They characterized several stages of progress in this skill over the early years. Yet embedded in this description is another description, that of what a more experienced person did to arrange the situation in order to reveal as much as possible about a child's skill at tying knots. Read the following description of the methodology Piaget and Inhelder used and take note of the behavior of the adult experimenter. It is similar to the type of graduated assistance discussed throughout this chapter as providing support for the development of problem-solving skills.

> The technique employed is simple in its extreme. To start with, the child is shown an ordinary simple knot tied tightly and asked to state what it is. . . . He is then asked to make a similar knot. If the child cannot tie a knot he is asked to form one round a thick stick or bobbin and his method of learning is studied. If he cannot succeed in this after a few attempts a knot is formed slowly whilst he watches and he is then asked to imitate the action he sees. If this also fails he is shown a piece of string in two colors (half blue, half red) and the process is explained as a story ("the red goes underneath, then on top, then inside, etc.") as the action gradually unfolds, after which he is invited to do the same. (pp. 105–106)

Although Piaget and Inhelder documented children's age-related skill at tying knots, they never did explain *how* children learn to tie knots. This is a familiar story in research on cognitive development. We now have substantial understanding of children's age-related progress in various cognitive domains but limited understanding of the factors that contribute to the development of these skills or the mechanisms that set them in place. Let's examine tying knots as a case in point.

Early in life children have experience watching others tie knots. They may watch someone tie shoelaces or tie two strings together to bind a package. As parents and others tie knots in a child's presence, especially when they are doing something for the child like tying his or her shoes, the more experienced partner may make some running commentary about the activity—commentary that serves as a prelude of things to come. One day, not too far off, the child will be taught to tie a knot, perhaps in his or her shoelaces. Of course, this learning will not occur in an instant but gradually, and all types of "knotty" circumstances may be met along the way: knots that are not knots at all but simply twisted laces or knots that are tied so tightly they will never be unknotted. Eventually, the child's knots will come to resemble the knots and bows that mother and father make, a real accomplishment for the young child. After all, it is not easy to take two thin flexible stings and arrange them so that they will stay joined—no less to do this when one's fine motor skills are in the process of developing.

As this description suggests, it is difficult to understand how skill at tying knots develops without paying some attention to the role that social partners play in the process. After children master their first knot—typically the overhand knot—most go on to tie more complex knots. They may do so largely on their own as they play with string and cord or as they try to model knots depicted in drawings. Sometimes more complex knots are taught to children, for example, in scouting where children study knots to get a merit badge or in sailing where children learn to tie knots in ropes in order to rig the sails. In these cases, various social mechanisms of explanation and instruction may come into play, including modeling, demonstration, instruction, and guided participation. My point is that from early on, children's developing skills in spatial representation and motor coordination coalesce in the everyday practice of tying knots, and more experienced people guide children through this learning process. Although Piaget and Inhelder (1956) provided insight into age-related changes in this skill, they did not consider the social context of how children learn to solve this particular type of problem. The goal of a sociocultural approach to problem solving is to understand and describe the social contributions to children's emerging problem-solving skills such as tying knots. More specifically, its purpose is to describe the role that social agents, both adults and other children, play in supporting and directing children's problem-solving skills.

WHAT IS PROBLEM SOLVING?

Every day people try to achieve many and varied goals. Some of these are modest, such as to have a good breakfast. Some are grand, such as to complete a long-term project at school or at work. In order to reach these goals, people engage in meaningful action, that is, people organize their actions in ways that are directed toward meeting their goals. The identification of an action goal and the delineation of steps or means to reach this goal is called *problem solving*. Problem solving is a central feature of human intelligence. In fact, some psychologists equate problem solving with thinking. An important feature of problem solving is overcoming obstacles that interfere with reaching the desired goal. Thus, problem solving involves a goal and one or more obstacles that need to be overcome to reach this goal.

What interests many cognitive researchers about problem solving is that it is a higher level mental function that is action-based and cognitively complex. That is, it is a purposeful, integrated aspect of human thinking that occurs during complex, voluntary, intelligent action. The term *integrated* refers to the fact that in order to solve a problem, a person uses many cognitive skills, including perception, memory, concepts, and perhaps language or other symbolic processes, like mathematics. Problem-solving skills are increasingly important as children get older and partake in more complex activities. Such activities typically present children with a problem or several problems to solve. Many of these activities, especially for young children, occur in social company. Thus, the social nature of problem solving and the role that social experience plays in the development of problem-solving skills are important to understand.

Developmental research on problem solving has concentrated on the emergence of certain critical components of this cognitive process. Of particular interest are how children understand or encode the problems they are trying to solve, the strategies that children have available to help them do this and how they choose particular strategies, and, finally, the role that content knowledge or expertise plays in problem solving and its development. These three aspects of problem solving develop over the years of childhood. As children get older, they encode more features of a problem, they get better at encoding features useful for solving a particular problem, and they allocate their attention more effectively during encoding (Siegler, 1976). A sociocultural approach addresses whether experience solving problems with other people influences what children encode and seeks to discover how children encode problem information. Developmental research has also shown that as children get older they are more likely to use strategies that help them solve problems and that children become increasingly skilled in using these strategies (Bjorkland, 1990). From a sociocultural perspective, a related issue concerns the role that the social world may play in children's selection and use of problem-solving strategies. Finally, current developmental research on the knowledge base asks whether prior knowledge enhances or biases children's problem solving (Chi, 1978; Penner & Klahr, 1996) and how knowledge is related to strategy use in different domains (Kuhn, Garcia-Mila, Zohar, & Andersen, 1995). From the vantage point of sociocultural theory, the issue is how social experience guides children in the formulation and use of knowledge to solve problems. The research described below addresses all these issues. It suggests that the social world makes critical contributions over the course of childhood to each of these important aspects of problem solving.

SOCIAL INTERACTION AND THE DEVELOPMENT OF PROBLEM SOLVING

Ben, age 4, shuffles into the family room with a jar of pennies that he has been saving. He announces to his mother that he wants to count them to see how much money he has. With mother looking on, Ben dumps the coins on the coffeetable and begins to count the pennies, one by one. All is going well until he counts some pennies a second time. Mother interrupts and suggests that he put the pennies in rows so that he doesn't count any twice. Ben agrees and begins to do this, but he aligns his rows poorly. Mother shows him how to straighten them by making a few sample rows herself. She also tells him that it is important to put 10 coins in each row and no more. They finish building the rows together and then they count the pennies: there are 47. A few days later Ben tells his mother that his father gave him some more pennies so he needs to count them again. Mother looks on as Ben dumps the pennies onto the coffeetable and begins, on his own, to set up rows of 10.

Children, even very young children, have the capability to respond to and interact with other people in the course of goal-directed action. According to Bruner (1982), shared intentional action, what I refer to here as *joint problem solving*, is at the heart of the socialization process.

Adults use many types of behaviors to encourage children's participation in joint problem solving, including modeling, instructing, scaffolding, and guided participation. Children use some of these same behaviors when they solve problems with age mates. Through shared activity children have the opportunity to learn about and practice problem-solving skills.

This chapter discusses joint problem solving in two types of social situations: adult–child and child–child interactions. Both have been the object of much research and both appear to benefit children's learning, at least under certain conditions. Throughout this discussion, I address the components of problem solving, namely, encoding, strategy acquisition and choice, and content knowledge, that appear to benefit from these interactions. Next I examine certain social factors that may influence how these transactions proceed. Characteristics of the child, the partner, the dyad, and the activity can affect how joint problem solving occurs and help determine what children learn from these experiences.

Adult–Child Problem Solving

Infancy

Even in the first year of life, children are involved with other people in activities that psychologists readily identify as joint problem solving. For instance, Rogoff, Malkin, and Gilbride (1984) observed adults as they interacted individually with one of two (fraternal) twin infants. These observations were conducted over a 13-month period, when the children were between 4 and 17 months of age. During this time the dyads played with different toys. I will concentrate on their interactions using a jack-in-the-box toy in which a bunny popped out of the container.

One way in which the adults engaged the infants in playing with the jack-in-the-box and supported the infants' learning about this toy was by organizing and managing subcomponents or subgoals of the activity. The adult's support changed over the course of the observations, as the infants matured and as they built up experience with the adults and with the toy. Early on, when the infants were 4 months old, the adults concentrated on maintaining the infants' attention to the toy, via the process called *joint attention* discussed in Chapter 4. When the infants were between 5½ and 12 months of age, the adults and infants displayed more mutual use of the toy, or *joint involvement* (Schaffer, 1992). Sometimes this was initiated by the adult and sometimes it was initiated by the infant. For example, one baby initiated joint involvement by staring at the toy and pushing it toward the adult when he was not playing with it. Even in these early interactions, some of the comments made by the adults suggest that they were trying to instruct the children about strategies, as the following comment illustrates. As one adult turned the handle of the toy, she said to the child: "And this makes him come out" (p. 39). Finally, when the infants were 12 to 17 months of age, the joint activity shifted to an emphasis on *joint management* of the social relations and their connection to the play. For instance, the baby would look at the adult, who would return the gaze, just before the bunny popped out.

Like Piaget, Rogoff and colleagues (1984) conclude that babies are active seekers of information. However, they add to this the observation that more experienced partners are a common and informative part of the everyday environment in which infants learn about the world. Thus, the active efforts that babies make to seek information about the world are heavily invested in obtaining information from the social context. By seeking information from others, babies learn important things about the world more generally and about problem solving in particular. This information includes where to direct their attention and how to manipulate objects to reach their goals. These types of transactions also provide infants with practice in the interpersonal aspects of such exchanges. Because these interactions are calibrated by the adult to the developmental needs of the infant, their effectiveness in helping the infant participate in and learn from the joint activity is enhanced.

Play contexts are not the only types of interactions involving infants and adults in which joint problem solving occurs. During routine activities, like mealtime, infants are engaged in practical activities that involve all types of problem solving, and parents and other adults are there to guide the infants through these experiences. Valsiner (1984) observed 28 infants between 10 and 15 months of age as they ate a meal with the assistance of a parent. The focus of these observations was who controlled the spoon, with particular attention to when and how control of the spoon shifted from parent to child. As the infants got older, they gradually took on more of the actions, like picking up the food on the spoon, moving the spoon through the air, guiding the spoon to the mouth, and getting the food into the mouth. Again, adults managed the children's entry into each of these behaviors, or subgoals, by scaffolding the children's actions, for example, by holding the spoon as the child did an action and then by letting the child do it on his or her own when the child was deemed ready to do so.

Five important characteristics of the social context of cognitive development are already evident in these early social interactions:

1. Both adult and child are actively engaged in activities that require thinking on both their parts.
2. Both adult and child assume some responsibility for the activity.
3. Adults help the child by dividing the task into subgoals and supporting the child's participation in these smaller, more manageable units of the problem.
4. Adult–child transactions change as children develop and become capable of managing more aspects of the problem on their own.
5. Adults assist children in the use of rudimentary strategies, such as how to maneuver the handle of the jack-in-the-box to release the bunny or how to navigate the spoon to the mouth.

These characteristics describe cognitive development as both an individual and a social process. From the first year of life, intellectual change is derived from the communion of the child's emerging capabilities with the adult's guidance and support. These interactions occur in the child's zone of proximal development (Vygotsky, 1978), or region of sensitivity for learning and growth.

Toddlerhood

Social influences on problem solving blossom during the second year as children's emerging skill with language takes on an increasingly important role. During this time, when children are in the one-word stage of language development, mothers often try to elicit from children a response that indicates the child's understanding. This process not only fosters early language learning, it connects words and their referents in the context of meaningful, goal-directed action. In other words, these interactions are embedded in a rudimentary form of joint problem solving.

Research by Greenfield (1984) illustrates this process. She describes an incident in which a mother handed her son, who was early in his second year, a toy telephone and asked "D'ya wanna call Daddy?" (p. 123). After several demonstrations by the mother as to how to use the telephone along with suggestions by mother for the child to phone daddy, the child uttered an unintelligible sound while the mother held the phone to his ear. What did the mother do next? She responded by saying, "Uh huh. Hello Daddy. Hello Daddy" (p. 123). Here, a shared activity that is structured largely by the adult but relies on the cooperation, interest, and participation of the child, eventually leads to the incorporation of the child's verbalization into a goal-directed and meaningful action by the child.

A recent study involving mothers and children in the second year suggests that such transactions benefit children in many domains of cognitive development (Gelman, Coley, Rosengren, Hartman, & Pappas, 1998). In addition to aiding language development and giving children experience at integrating language and problem solving, adult–child interaction can enhance concept development, an area in which there is much growth during early childhood. Concept development is the foundation of the developing knowledge base, and therefore is instrumental in supporting the development of problem-solving skills. What is interesting in the research by Gelman and colleagues is its description of the emergence in social context of this critical part of the knowledge base.

Gelman and colleagues (1998) observed children between 20 and 35 months of age as they read a picture book with their mothers. The mothers made many different types of statements about objects and features of the world that provided opportunities for children to learn new concepts. The conceptual information that the mothers conveyed was of a particular sort. In these interactions, mothers tended to direct children's attention to whole objects (e.g., balls), not parts of objects. They also made statements about object identity ("That's an aardvark"), the relations of objects to one another ("That's a desk. That's a desk, too."), general information about objects ("Bats live in caves"), and even sometimes told children about categories that are complex or richly structured ("Did you know that when a pig gets to be big they're called hogs?") (p. 125). Although it is unknown how children interpret these statements, the fact that natural discourse between mothers and children as young as 20 months of age includes information of this breadth and complexity suggests that this type of social context can be a rich source of information for children's developing knowledge base. Even though adults provide much of the content and structure in these interactions, the child's contribution to the process should not be overlooked. Mothers were able to tailor their comments to the child's level of understanding because children communicated their understanding by showing interest and acknowledging information that made sense to them.

The guidance provided by adults when children are toddlers supports the development of children's problem solving in many ways. It directs the child's attention in new learning contexts to particular aspects of the situation and to ways of encoding incoming information. It also helps build the child's knowledge base, which is essential to problem solving and its development.

Early Childhood

Much of the research investigating how adult–child interaction relates to problem solving has included adults, typically parents, and children between 3 and 5 years of age. This age range is particularly amenable to this topic for several reasons. First, at this age children are quite competent with language and communication, which are important structural features of social–cognitive transactions involving adults and children. Second, much development in a wide range of cognitive domains is occurring at this time. Third, despite impressive cognitive changes, preschoolers are still very young, and are therefore in the company of older people much of the time. This social "co-incidence" provides substantial opportunity for more experienced individuals to direct and guide children's everyday problem solving.

Early childhood, the period that Fraiberg (1959) called the "magic years," is when children wonder about everything, especially the world in which they live. Many of their questions begin with "why" and "how." Callanan and Oakes (1992) asked parents of 3-, 4-, and 5-year-old children to keep diaries over a 2-week period of their children's "why" and "how" questions. The researchers were interested in many features of these conversations, including their frequency, the topics children covered, the form of speech children used, and the types of explanations parents provided in response to these questions. They found, as every parent knows, that the frequency of these questions increased over these years. Interestingly, at all of these ages "why" and "how" questions tended to be complex, that is, children rarely asked about the world by just stating "Why" or "How." Rather, their questions included referents, ideas, and observations—for example, Why is the sky blue? or How does the telephone know which house to call? Most of these types of questions arose during shared activity with the parent rather than being introduced by the child when the parent and child were not jointly engaged. Finally, parents' explanations often contained information about mechanisms, that is, how the world works, as the following exchange illustrates:

> CHILD: Where does the rain come from?
>
> PARENT: First the water collects in the clouds, then they get really filled . . . (p. 222n)

For children as young as 4 years of age, more than half of the parents' conversational turns provided a causal explanation.

These results tell us several things about cognitive development during this period. First, they indicate that parents regularly provide children with information about the world and about how things in the world work. This type of experience helps shape children's growing knowledge base, which is critical to the development of problem solving. Second, these data confirm the view that children actively seek knowledge and that their understanding of the world often emerges in the flow of interaction with more experienced partners. Third, these observations suggest some of the unique opportunities available to children in everyday social interaction for the development of skills that are important to problem solving. I use the word *unique* here to emphasize the fact that these types of opportunities for cognitive growth are socially dynamic and constructed. As a result, they are not available in contexts that do not involve social interaction.

In order to better understand how social interaction with adults may lead to cognitive growth, Wood and colleagues (Wood, Bruner, & Ross, 1976; Wood & Middleton, 1975; Wood, Wood, & Middleton, 1978) conducted a series of studies. In this research, the investigators introduced, outlined, and demonstrated the process of *scaffolding*, which is one type of adult–child interaction that supports children's cognitive growth. Scaffolding occurs when an adult in the course of solving a problem with a child assumes responsibility for arranging and managing the activity so that the child can participate at a level *just beyond* his or her current capabilities. As a result, scaffolding supports the child's interaction in the zone of proximal development. The adult, acting on information obtained from the child, creates a situation that allows the child to concentrate on aspects of the task that are within his or her grasp. The child can then learn about the task by participating in it and experiencing a sense of accomplishment at its conclusion.

A critical feature of scaffolding is that it is adjusted over the course of a problem-solving interaction to accommodate the child's changing degree of skill and confidence. The child's actions clue the adult about the level of intervention or support that the child needs, and the adult then uses this information to modify his or her subsequent contribution in the interaction in a process called *contingent responding*. If the child is doing well, the adult can provide less support than he or she did in the immediately preceding exchange. If the child is floundering, the adult may need to provide more support.

To study in more detail how the process works, Wood and Middleton (1975) observed 12 mother–child dyads as they constructed a pyramid made of wooden blocks. The children, who were 3 to 4 years of age, initially played with the blocks on their own, then they interacted with their mothers in building the pyramid, and finally each child constructed the pyramid on his or her own. To characterize the nature of the mothers' responses, the researchers divided the interaction into a series of episodes and then coded each of the mothers' interactional turns according to a five-level, hierarchical sequence. These represented different levels of intervention or support by the mother and ranged from general instructions, which were the least regulating in terms of assisting or guiding the child's actions, to manipulation of the task materials in specific goal-directed ways, which was the most regulating. The five levels were:

1. General verbal instruction.
2. Specific verbal instruction.
3. Mother shows the child which materials to use.
4. Mother provides the child with the materials to use and prepares the materials for assembly.
5. Mother demonstrates an operation, such as selecting and assembling the materials, as the child looks on.

To gauge the effectiveness of maternal instruction in the interactional flow, Wood and Middleton identified whether the child succeeded or failed in his or her problem-solving attempts in the step immediately following the instruction. They also examined maternal response contingencies and the child's performance on the independent trial following the interaction. They found, first of all, that mothers did respond contingently to their children's actions during joint problem solving. Mothers actively adjusted their level of assistance in relation to the child's needs, which the researchers called *the child's region of sensitivity* as indexed by the child's performance in the immediately preceding episode. In an ideal contingent relation, mothers would either increase the help they provided after the child was unsuccessful on a turn or they would decrease their level of assistance following success by the child on a turn.

Wood and Middleton observed individual differences among the mothers in their patterns of contingent responding. This permitted examination of the effectiveness of the different types of responding. Some mothers had high rates of contingent responding, whereas others had low rates. In support of the hypothesis that contingent responding aids learning, the researchers found that mothers who had higher rates had children who performed better on the solitary posttest than mothers with lower rates. It is important to emphasize that the total amount of instruction that mothers provided did not relate to the child's later task performance: only the mothers' sensitive use of scaffolding did.

In an effort to clarify the causal relations in these findings, Wood, Wood, and Middleton (1978) conducted a follow-up study that involved a trained experimenter working with children of this same age on the same task. Children were taught to construct the pyramid by the experimenter, who used either a contingent approach, a verbal–didactic approach, physical demonstration, or a combination of verbal encouragement and demonstration. The research team found that children instructed with the contingent approach did better on the later independent trial than children instructed in any of the other three ways. Incidentally, verbal–didactic instruction was the least effective, perhaps because it was not informed by, and therefore calibrated to, the children's changing needs over the course of the interaction.

The main conclusion that can be drawn from these studies is that adults are capable of providing contingent responses to children's immediate cognitive needs during joint problem solving. When adults do this, it benefits children's learning. Now that we know it is useful, we need to know if and when it occurs. To what extent do parents provide such guidance for their children? To answer this question, Pacifici and Bearison (1991) observed adults and 2½- to 3½-year-old children as they worked on a puzzle together. Some dyads included mothers and other dyads included an experimenter who was trained to provide ideal contingent responses tailored to the child's skill and immediate learning needs. Like Wood and his colleagues, these investigators devised a coding scheme that identified the mother's instructions in terms of how explicit they were in addressing the child's immediate learning needs. A response was identified as *contingent* if it was less explicit following a correct response by the child and more explicit following an incorrect response. To assess children's learning, an individual posttest followed the interaction.

What did the investigators find? Mothers did respond contingently to their children, but they did so at less than the ideal rate (with the ideal rate being defined as one that was consistently and contingently provided to the child's needs). In addition, although children who worked with mothers showed some improvement from the pretest to the posttest, those who worked with the experimenter during the "ideal" interaction had better posttest scores than children who worked with mothers. These results are consistent with those of Wood and Middleton (1975). They show that mothers sometimes responded contingently to their young children during joint problem solving and when they did it benefited learning. The results also suggest that all parent-child dyads are not the same in terms of the cognitive interactions they experience. Later in the chapter, certain characteristics of the social context of joint cognitive activity are suggested as explanations for the different patterns observed in the mother–child dyads. For now, the discussion builds on the concept of scaffolding by focusing on the different ways in which adults support children's learning in early childhood.

Saxe, Guberman, and Gearhart (1987) observed mothers and 2½- to 4½-year-old children as they played number games together. Mothers helped the children by directing their attention to critical features of the problem situation—for example, during one counting game a mother said "This dot is next" as she pointed to the next item to count. Mothers also offered strategic assistance—for example, mothers would tell their children to count the dots in rows. Contributions to the developing knowledge base also occurred, as in questions like "What number is this?" and "What number comes after 5?" Consider the following interactional exchange as an example of how these various types of information may be woven together as adults and young children solve problems together.

MOTHER: Count the dots.

CHILD: (*Recites "1" through "6" correctly while haphazardly pointing to dots.*)

MOTHER: Start over and this time count the dots in rows.

CHILD: (*Correctly counts the bottom row and continues to count "5, 6, 8" while pointing to the first, second, and third dots in the second row.*)

MOTHER: No, what comes after 6?

CHILD: Eleven.

MOTHER: Seven comes after 6.

In this example, it is clear how the mother's instruction is tailored to the child's needs and is structured according to the subgoal of the problem on which the dyad is working. By breaking a problem into subgoals and focusing their assistance and instruction in these areas, adults demonstrate that a problem can be divided into parts and that these parts can be operated on individually in order to reach the overall goal—an understanding that is essential to the development and use of problem-solving skills.

Research suggests that the process of encoding may be of particular focus in the social–cognitive experiences that children have in early childhood. Wertsch, McNamee, McLane, and Budwig (1980) observed 2½-, 3½-, and 4½-year-old children as they worked with their mothers on a puzzle. The completed puzzle was supposed to look exactly like a model puzzle that was presented to the dyad at the outset of the session. The researchers were particularly interested in what the child looked at and who regulated the child's eye gazes. Gazes were labeled as *other-regulated* when the child gazed following a mother's gesturing or reference to the model or puzzle pieces. For example, McLane (1981) observed the following comment by a mother:

> MOTHER: What's the (*mother points to yellow square on model*) color (*3½-year-old child looks at model*) in the bottom corner? (*Child looks at copy, then at pieces.*) (p. 68)

Gazes were identified as *self-regulated* when they did not follow some guidance by mother.

The investigators observed that over these years, children's gazes at the problem-solving materials shifted from other- to self-regulated. They also found that when younger children looked at the model puzzle, regardless of whether their gaze was self- or other-regulated, they were less able than older children to extract information relevant to puzzle completion. Did working with mother help younger children develop or refine this skill? The data suggest that working with an adult provides children with opportunities to develop this skill. Specifically, mothers tended to make comments following children's placement errors that directed children's attention to features of the model that were important to the part of the puzzle that they were working on, as the following case illustrates:

> MOTHER: (*after 3½-year-old child has misplaced a square*) I think (*as she points to model*) you have to (*child looks at model*) check (*child looks at copy, removes misplaced piece, places it correctly*) over here. (*Mother finishes pointing, child looks at model.*) Ta dum! (McLane, 1981, p. 57)

This type of exchange suggests that opportunities for the development and refinement of encoding skills, which are central to problem solving, are part of adult–child joint problem solving in early childhood.

The literature reviewed so far suggests that joint problem solving involving adults and children in the preschool years may affect children's skill at encoding problem information and their knowledge base. Is there any evidence that adult–child interaction during this developmental period benefits children's strategy use? A study conducted by Freund (1990) that used a sorting and classification task suggests that strategy development in this period can be positively affected by problem solving with an adult. Dyads composed of 3- or 5-year-old children and their mothers were observed as they sorted miniature furniture and placed these in rooms in a dollhouse. After the interaction, children participated in an individual posttest that involved sorting and placing similar items. The assistance that mothers provided during the

interaction was identified either as *low level,* that is, it included primarily item-specific comments and little strategy information; or as *high
level,* which included strategy information useful for solving the problem, namely, how to group the items. Children whose mothers provided assistance that was predominantly high level were more accurate
in how they grouped the items on the posttest than children whose
mothers provided low-level assistance. This suggests that preschool-age
children can learn about strategies for solving problems from exposure
to adult strategy use during joint problem solving.

All of the research discussed above was conducted in the laboratory. Is there evidence from outside the lab that social interaction between adults and children can provide opportunities for the development of children's problem-solving skills? Gelman, Massey, and
McManus (1991) observed parents and young children as they explored specially designed exhibits at a children's museum. One of the
exhibits involved counting. The display was fitted with signs that identified the exhibit ("Counting Box") and had written directions explaining
how to play the game. Because preschoolers were unable to read the
directions, the investigators were interested in whether the adults ac-
companying the children would seize the opportunity to instruct the
children.

The researchers observed that only one-third of the adults who accompanied the children actually read the sign to the children and only
one-fifth of the adults encouraged the children to do the activity. However, when adults read the signs and encouraged the children to do the
activity, children were more likely to engage in it than when this information was not provided. Consistent with laboratory findings, when
adults direct children's attention to a problem or activity and define
the goals for them, children's opportunity to learn is enhanced. However, the results also suggest that even when adults are able to scaffold
children's learning, they may not choose to do so.

A second set of observations by this same research team (Gelman
et al., 1991) examined a related question: Does input from the social
world need to be "face-to-face" in order for it to benefit children's
learning? To study this issue, the researchers used a museum exhibit
equipped with a computer and speakers that presented and explained
the exhibit in scientific terms to the children. Preschoolers were
observed playing with this exhibit before and after the computer was
installed. Before it was installed, few children—in fact, only one child—
ever used the exhibit in a way that demonstrated any scientific understanding. But after the computer was installed, two-thirds of the
children demonstrated such understanding. What does this research
tell us? Information about how to solve problems comes in many

forms. Some of it comes from the task itself, some comes from social agents, and some comes from tools introduced by the social world to aid children's problem solving. These results indicate that face-to-face explanation is not a necessary condition for learning. Of course, we cannot forget that the input from the computer was designed and staged by other more experienced individuals—which is a specialized form of social interaction.

Research on adult–child interaction during the preschool years, a time of marked expansion in the range of cognitive problems within children's grasp, is accompanied by a change in the cognitive assistance that adults provide for children during joint problem solving. Guidance is now more fluidly integrated with and reliant upon language. However, nonverbal assistance continues to play an important role, as research on eye gaze indicates. Processes of social interaction that appear to benefit cognitive growth, specifically contingent responding, are similar to those observed during the years of infancy and toddlerhood. There is some evidence that children's skill at encoding and strategy use, along with the developing knowledge base, are influenced by social interaction in the years of early childhood. Further study of the causal connections between specific aspects of cognitive development and the social context of problem solving is needed.

Middle Childhood

There has been less research on parent–child problem solving involving children in the years of middle childhood. (This is not true in all aspects of problem solving, however. As we will see in the next chapter, research on social influences on the development of children's planning skills concentrates rather heavily on the years of middle childhood.) It is also the case that much of the research on social influences on problem solving during middle childhood concentrates on peer interaction and teacher–child interaction. This reflects the fact that during middle childhood children's social lives change dramatically, and therefore children's opportunity to develop cognitive skills in social context also changes. Children spend more time with other children, mostly age mates. Because children of this age are under less continuous adult supervision, most of their peer experiences occur outside of adult range. Furthermore, children's contact with adults outside the family, especially teachers, increases substantially in the years of middle childhood.

One study (discussed in Chapter 4) on the development of memory in social context is relevant to the present discussion on the development of problem-solving skills in social context. This research examined adult–child interaction as mothers worked with their 7-year-old children on a sorting and classification task (Rogoff & Gauvain, 1986). Recall children were tested after their mothers taught them how to group 18 familiar household items into six categories. On the basis of their performance on the posttest, children were identified as either low, intermediate, or high scorers. These groups were then examined in relation to the type of cognitive assistance mothers provided during the joint session, especially the types of problem-solving strategies used. Low scorers were not to any great degree exposed to the correct organization or grouping of the items during the interaction and their participation in deciding how to sort the items during the interaction was minimal. High scorers received the most guidance about the correct organization of the items and their category labels and these children participated to a large extent in the sorting decisions that were made during the interaction. Intermediate scorers had moderate levels of exposure to the category labels and moderate levels of participation. These results are similar to those found in the earlier years of childhood, and indicate that children's participation in a social context in which strategies that are useful for solving a problem increases the likelihood that children will use these strategies in later individual performance on these same types of tasks.

Because children's social learning opportunities in middle childhood expand to include teachers, researchers have compared the cognitive assistance provided by parents with that provided by adults who have been trained as teachers. This research shows that teachers and parents contribute differently to children's experience during interactions involving joint problems solving. In a study with 6-year-old children, Wertsch, Minick, and Arns (1984) compared adult–child interaction with the children's mothers and with elementary school teachers. The dyads worked on a construction task together that involved copying a three-dimensional model of a toy barnyard. The researchers studied how the various problem-solving behaviors needed to accomplish the task were performed by the partners: specifically, who looked at the model, who picked up the pieces, and who placed the pieces. They found an interesting difference between the assistance provided by mothers and that provided by teachers. Mothers were more likely than teachers to perform these three problem-solving behaviors when they worked with the children, whereas children who worked with teachers did more of these problem-solving behaviors on their own.

This difference may be due to the different levels of education that the mothers and teachers had. The mothers in this study had fewer years of schooling than the teachers. Education has been found to be an influential factor in maternal instruction (Laosa, 1980). The mothers and teachers may also have had different goals when they solved the problems with the children. In other research on mother–children problem solving, Renshaw and Gardner (1990) found that most mothers adopt a learning goal rather than a performance goal when working with their children. A learning goal is associated with indirect teaching methods, including fewer regulating behaviors like checking, monitoring, and evaluation. The adults also had different relationships with the children, which also could have influenced the nature of the transactions (Gauvain & DeMent, 1991). Finally, teachers have specialized training, and this surely influences how they interact with children during joint problem solving. We now turn to a study that focused on social interaction and children's learning with a teacher to explore in more detail how teachers may support the development of problem-solving skills.

Palinscar and Brown (1984) were interested in devising an instructional program that would help children who have difficulty comprehending what they read. The approach they developed, which is called *reciprocal instruction,* is based on Vygotsky's (1978) notion of the zone of proximal development. Reciprocal instruction supports children's learning by helping children participate in reading comprehension activities that they are unable to do when they read on their own. For example, a lesson based on this approach initially involves the students and the teacher as they read a paragraph aloud. Then the teacher uses questions and examples to help the children learn how to extract meaning from the text. The teacher may begin by summarizing the main point of the paragraph, then he or she guides the children through an examination of the content of the paragraph, focusing especially on passages that need clarification. At the end of the lesson the teacher prompts the students to anticipate what will come next. Through these graduated steps, the teacher demonstrates strategies for examining text, such as summarizing, clarifying, and predicting.

Research on this approach indicates that it does help students learn to read more strategically, and thereby enhances reading comprehension. The average reading comprehension score of the seventh-grade children in this research before reciprocal instruction was 20% correct. After the instruction the children's reading comprehension averaged 80% correct—and this improvement was evident 6 months after the instruction (Palinscar, Brown, & Campione, 1993). Other research has demonstrated the effectiveness of this approach with individuals whose comprehension scores range from low to average and with children as young as fourth graders and older than seventh graders (Rosenshine & Meister, 1994, summarize these results). These findings support the general claim that solving problems with an experienced partner who targets cognitive assistance to the learner's needs can aid the development of problem solving in a particular domain. They also support the specific claim that the strategies that children use during social participation increase the likelihood that the children will use these same strategies later on their own.

In sum, research on adult–child problem solving at different points in development reveals a consistent picture. Children are involved with more experienced partners for a very large portion of their daily lives, and these experiences often involve solving problems. There are strong indications in the research that during these interactions adults assist children in the development and use of many of the skills critical for solving problems, in particular, encoding, strategy use, and content knowledge. This does not mean that these skills originate in social interaction, though they sometimes may. Research testing this specific hypothesis has yet to be done. But research does suggest that social interaction with adults is an important source of input for children during the years in which they are developing and refining their problem-solving skills. More research is needed to pin down how specific areas of cognitive development may benefit from problem solving with adults, as well as to delineate more precisely what factors contribute to the success or failure of these transactions.

Child–Child Problem Solving

Research on adult–child problem solving reflects Vygotsky's view that the guidance and support that occurs when children work with more experienced partners may serve as mechanisms of cognitive growth. In contrast, the Piagetian view stresses the role of cognitive conflict between partners who are closely but not identically matched in their understanding as a mechanism of individual development. From this perspective, a near-intellectual partner possessing a slightly more sophisticated understanding is the person best suited to providing intellectual impetus for growth. Although these two perspectives differ in their views on what particular arrangement of partners best facilitates cognitive growth, the main idea, that peer interaction can promote cognitive development, was proposed by both theorists (Tudge & Rogoff, 1989).

One important way in which adult–child and peer problem solving differ is when in the child's life they begin. Whereas adult–child problem solving appears in the first year, peer problem solving comes later. How much later? Brownell and Carriger (1991) studied the early development of peer problem solving by examining the emergence of skills that are needed for this process to occur, that is, the precursors of peer cognitive interaction. These researchers observed dyads of same-age children between the ages of 12 and 30 months. The dyads were presented with a problem that required cooperation in order to be solved. Several problem versions were used, though all involved a similar goal, which was to place small toys in a cup. In order to reach this goal, an action was required, such as pushing a lever or rotating a handle, and an obstacle, a barrier, was in place. What did the children do on these tasks? None of the 12 month olds solved the problem. Though they manipulated the materials in an effort to solve the problem, they were unable to coordinate their actions to reach the goal. Half of the 18 month olds solved the problem, but when they were presented with similar problems following success, they were unable to repeat it. All of the 24- and 30-month-old children solved the problem, and they did so multiple times.

There are several observations of interest here. First, all of the children were engaged in actions that could be called problem solving. That is, they manipulated the materials in ways that indicated some attempt to solve the problem. However, only the older children were able to coordinate their actions to reach the goal. Second, one important behavior of the older, but not younger, children that contributed to learning in social context was watching the partner's behaviors, a process Brownell and Carriger (1991) called *monitoring*. Although the rate of monitoring was equivalent for the 18-, 24-, and 30-month-olds, the older children were more likely to watch their partner when he or she was engaged in problem solving. Thus, it is not social attention per se but selective social attention to particular actions by the partner that is critical. These findings also suggest that very young children may face much difficulty in managing the various demands of a joint problem-solving activity. To illustrate, Table 6.1 shows the age-related patterns in the toddlers' monitoring of one another during this task. Notice that monitoring when both children were engaged with the task increases with child age. For Brownell and Carriger, this suggests that the older children were trying to establish joint task-related efforts. In contrast, younger children were more likely than older children to look at the other child when only one of the children was on task. This suggests that younger children were monitoring one another more for social than for task reasons.

It appears the younger children had greater difficulty in managing the multiple demands of joint activity. The social, cognitive, and emotional demands of joint engagement may compete or collide in such early peer interactions, and as a result these may disrupt the problem-solving activity and the chance for children to learn from the experience. Furthermore, some aspects of problem solving in social context

TABLE 6.1. Mean Frequency That Toddlers Monitored (or Looked at) Partner during Solution Attempts

Monitoring behavior	Age of child		
	18 months	24 months	30 months
Monitor— Both on task	6.30	7.40	8.30
Monitor— One on task	4.70	3.40	1.70

Note. From Brownell and Carriger (1991). Copyright 1991 by the American Psychological Association. Adapted by permission.

may take precedence at certain ages. As these data suggest, the social aspects of joint cognitive activity, rather than the cognitive aspects, may be of more interest and concern to very young children. With increasing age, children pay more attention to the problem-solving efforts of other people. This may be a valuable learning tool in that it can provide children with information about the important features or actions in a problem-solving context. In many ways it is a form of social referencing, though what is being sought (or referenced) is cognitive information and not emotional information, which is typically the object of study in research on social referencing. In sum, these data indicate that children as young as 2 years of age can collaborate in certain circumstances with other children in order to solve a problem. Thus, some of the social skills required for joint problem solving are already starting to appear by this young age. Furthermore, children of this age are able in simple problem-solving situations to adjust their own actions in relation to those of a partner in order to reach a shared goal. Brownell and Carriger believe that these age-related patterns relied, in good measure, on children's increasing competence in other areas important to joint problem solving, especially communication.

Communication skills are important for children to reap the cognitive benefits of peer interaction. Much change in communication skills occurs in the preschool years. Cooper (1980) observed same-age dyads composed of either 3½- or 4½-year-old children as they balanced blocks. She found better performance by the older dyads and concluded that this was directly related to these children's communicative skills. Older children were more responsive to their partner's questions, which means they shared knowledge useful for solving the problem. Dyads of older children also talked more about how to label the blocks in ways that aided problem solving, suggesting that their communication focused on strategic components of the task. Finally, dyads with older children used more attention-focusing statements, which may have influenced how children encoded the problem space and helped the partners devise a shared definition or understanding of the problem. All of these behaviors were related to more efficient and successful problem solving by the partners. This suggests that skills that develop with age, such as communicative competence, directly impact the nature of the transactions that children have with peers during joint problem solving. This, in turn, influences the opportunities that children have when working with peers that may be useful for the development of problem-solving skills.

The research reviewed so far suggests that peer interaction can play an important role in children's learning. But are two heads always better than one? Azmitia (1988) asked this question in a study that involved 5-year-old children who worked in pairs copying a model made of plastic building blocks. This research was concerned with the general question of whether peer interaction can aid learning, as well as with the more specific question of whether certain features of peer interaction promote learning more than other features. The feature of interest was expertise. Children participated in one of three conditions: (1) they worked alone, (2) they worked with a child who had the same ability as themselves on the task, or (3) they worked with a child of different ability on the task. The children had a solitary pretest and posttest in order to examine how these various social conditions related to children's learning.

Children who worked with a partner did better on the solitary posttest than those who worked alone. The benefits of collaboration were especially pronounced for children who were novices and were paired with children who were experts. What happened during these interactions that aided learning? The problem-solving behavior that distinguished novices and experts was looking at the model. Experts studied the model more than novices, indicating that they were encoding more features of the problem space. Interestingly, in same-ability dyads, experts watched each other more than novices watched each other. Thus, expert pairs studied the model and each other more than novice pairs did. What about mixed-ability dyads? When novices and experts were paired, the experts spent more time than the novices looking at the model. So what did the novices do? They watched the experts! And what they saw was someone who looked at the model—a lot.

Children's understanding of a task before they engage in joint activity may influence what happens when children work in groups involving children of same or mixed ability. Pine and Messer (1998) observed 5- to 7-year-old children as they worked on balance beam problems in groups of four that included children of either same- or mixed-ability levels. Before solving the problems on their own, the children observed the experimenter solve several balance beam problems. The children were then assigned either to a group identified as "discussion" or to a group identified as "no discussion." The discussion groups stayed together in their groups and talked about the balance beam problems. The no discussion groups went back to their classrooms and worked alone on these same problems. Children in the mixed-ability groups benefited more than children in same-ability groups from social experience, with one exception. Children who held to a "center theory," the view that everything balances in the middle of the beam (which is a rudimentary and not very strategic view of the task in that only a limited number of problems can be solved successfully from this understanding), were more resistant to input from others. For these children, their skill on the balance beam remained unchanged whether or not they discussed balance beam problems with other children. These results suggest that children respond differently to information from others depending on the understanding they bring to the joint activity. These results are consistent with those by Hawkins, Homolsky, and Heide (1984), who found that changes in children's competence from social experience may be limited to particular points or stages of skill acquisition.

These observations suggest that the opportunity to work with a peer of different expertise provides children, but especially children who are less experienced or skilled, with the chance to learn effective strategies by seeing them used, and used effectively, in the course of solving a problem. An interesting finding from the Azmitia (1988) study is that same-ability dyads, compared with dyads of mixed ability, had more discussion about strategy. However, in this research, talk about strategy was not related to children's learning from social interaction. This is interesting in relation to adult–child problem solving in which talk is a central structural feature. It appears that during peer interaction, at least in the early to middle years of childhood, opportunities to learn are largely rooted in chances to observe rather than to talk about a partner's behaviors.

This is a puzzling finding, especially given that other research (see, e.g., Cooper, 1980) indicates that increasing communicative competence among preschoolers is related to more effective joint problem solving among peers. To explore this issue further, Teasley (1995) examined whether the type of talk that is fairly common in adult–child interaction and that has been shown to be related to children's learning from social experience occurs when children in the years of middle childhood solve problems together. She also wondered whether, if such talk occurs, it benefits children's learning in the same way in peer interaction as it does in adult–child interaction. The type of talk Teasley studied is that which emphasizes task analysis and strategy. It includes explanations, inferences, arguments, goals, plans, and strategies. Teasley called this *interpretive talk,* which she distinguished from *descriptive talk,* which includes discussion of task elements but not higher level task analysis and strategy.

In this study, dyads of 10- to 11-year-old children worked on a computer task that involved scientific reasoning. They were asked to determine how a spaceship moved, and especially to discover the function of an unlabeled computer key, referred to as "the mystery key." Children worked in one of four social conditions: alone and encouraged to talk aloud, with a partner and encouraged to talk aloud, alone and asked not to talk aloud, and with a partner and asked not to talk aloud. These four conditions vary the extent and nature of verbal and social contact during joint problem solving and allow for closer examination of these processes.

Teasley found that the amount of talk in which children engaged, regardless of whether a child worked alone or with a partner, was related to success on the task. Also, the proportion of interpretive talk was positively related to performance and the proportion of descriptive talk was negatively related to performance. This research shows that certain types of verbalization are related to learning and suggests that the internal processing of information is different when children hear verbalizations about what they are doing. Perhaps in the course of verbalizing action, even when solving a problem alone, children may articulate or peruse ideas or thoughts that may not be considered mentally but may be helpful in learning about and solving the problem. For example, comments about motives ("Why am I doing this?") or inferences ("So why do these two fit together?") may be brought more into conscious awareness, and this may make them available for examination. These data do not confirm that this process is developmentally related. It is reasonable to hypothesize that with more experience solving problems, and with increasing age, that such verbalized comments may still occur, but that they may be likely to be in the form of self-talk. Although Luria (1961) argued that the verbal regulation of children's behavior undergoes developmental change from early to middle childhood (i.e., from verbal regulation by others, to verbalized regulation by the self, to internal self-talk or self-regulation), it is possible that on new and challenging tasks even older learners may engage in and benefit from verbalized regulation either by the self or by others. Teasley's research suggests that children in the later years of middle childhood may benefit from such talk.

Although these data suggest that verbalization by the self does benefit learning, do they also indicate that the presence of a partner provides any benefit for children's learning beyond that of verbalized self-talk? In this study, Teasley observed that children who worked in dyads that were encouraged to talk to each other produced more strategic or interpretive types of talk than children who worked in dyads that were asked not to talk. She also found that children who worked in dyads that were discouraged from talking had the lowest scores of any of the four groups. Apparently, one reason that collaboration aids learning is because it increases the likelihood that children will engage in the kinds of behaviors that support learning, like examining ideas and actions. Another lesson from this research cannot be ignored, however. Although interpretive talk is more likely when children work with a partner, working with a partner is no guarantee that it will occur. And the results suggest that if, for some reason, the partners do not engage in this kind of talk (e.g., they are instructed not to talk), working with a partner may be detrimental. The other important message in this research is that it is not the talk alone that matters: it is *what is talked about* that counts. Interpretive or strategic talk benefits learning and descriptive or low-level talk does not.

It is worth discussing the fact that Teasley's (1995) results, which stress verbal communication, and those of Azmitia (1988), which stress nonverbal communication, seem to contradict one another. However, they may be reconciled to some degree by remembering that the children in the two studies were of different ages. Perhaps verbal exchange plays an increasingly important role as children develop and become more skilled with using communication during problem solving with peers. This does not mean that verbalization does not occur among younger children. It does and, as Cooper's (1980) results show, it can benefit children's performance when they work together and talk about the problem. Across these various studies, different tasks were used; this, too, may have influenced both the frequency and utility of talk in peer interaction. For instance, learning with peers on computer-based tasks may be most aided by communication, whereas learning with peers on tasks that involve the physical manipulation of objects may be most aided by observation.

Other factors may also influence the likelihood of interpretive or strategic discussion among peers during joint problem solving. In particular, children's relationship to one another, such as their friendship, is important. This was shown in a study involving fifth graders (11½-year-olds) who worked with same-age partners on a task that involved scientific reasoning (Azmitia & Montgomery, 1993). Dyads were asked to determine which variable(s) made healthy plants sick. Children were paired with either a friend or with a classmate whom they knew but had not previously identified as either a close friend or as someone they disliked. A comparison of scores on the individual pretests and posttests showed that friends improved their performance following interaction more than acquaintances did. This may be explained by the fact that friends behaved differently from acquaintances during the collaborative session. Friends offered more explanations, elaborations, and critiques to each other than acquaintances did. In terms of strategy use, friends were more likely to justify their strategies and solution proposals, as well as to check and evaluate their solutions. Friends know more about each other than do acquaintances and strangers, and this may promote a different type of joint problem solving in dyads defined along this dimension. These findings suggest that during joint problem solving, friendship can benefit children's learning beyond what occurs when children work with peers who are not close friends. Thus, social relationships contribute in meaningful ways to the generation of communicative exchanges that regulate the cognitive opportunities that emerge in joint problem solving.

The evidence discussed thus far suggests that peer interaction can benefit learning. It is not clear, though, whether it is the interaction per se that matters or what the interaction contains, that is, the content that peers exchange. Recall that this same question surfaced in adult–child research and led to a study of whether face-to-face interaction was critical to the social–cognitive process (Gelman et al., 1991). Perhaps properly timed and informative feedback is sufficient to explain the benefits of peer interaction to children's cognitive development. To explore this question, Ellis, Klahr, and Siegler (1993) studied the effects of feedback and collaboration on children's learning, measured by the children's skill prior to and following the interaction. Their study focused on the domain of mathematics, specifically mathematical rules used to determine the relative values of pairs of decimal fractions. Each child solved a series of decimal problems in which he or she was asked which of two values was larger. Three social conditions were studied: children worked alone, with a partner who used the same rule, or with a partner who used a different rule. Each of these conditions was further divided into a "feedback" or a "no feedback" group. Feedback for those in the feedback group pertained to the correct answer and was provided to the child(ren) immediately following each problem. To obtain the feedback, the child(ren) pulled off a sticker covering the correct answer that was placed alongside the pair of numbers.

The investigators found that only the children who received feedback about the correctness of their answers improved their skill at solving decimal problems. Of the children who received feedback, those who worked with a partner, compared with those who worked alone, were twice as likely to improve. This indicates two points about social influences on cognitive development: one, feedback aids learning, and two, feedback in the presence of a partner enhances learning beyond receiving this same feedback when one works alone.

Further analyses of these data by Ellis (1995) looked more closely at the interactional processes in the dyads that may have led to differences in learning on this task. She found that children who generated correct strategies were likely to abandon them when their ideas were not met with interest by their partner. In contrast, children who received interest from their partners regarding their new ideas were likely to retain the correct strategy. Other social factors, like partner engagement and clarity of communication, also appear to increase the likelihood that new, correct strategies will be maintained from peer interaction.

In sum, peer interaction can be a context for individual learning and development. However, aspects of the interaction, such as relative expertise, the children's social relationship, and the availability and use of feedback, can all affect what is learned. It is clear that when problem solving occurs in a social setting, certain opportunities that can benefit learning may occur. In particular, the opportunity to elaborate or defend solutions and the chance to receive support as one tries out new or tentative strategies may enhance intellectual development in social context. Although peer interaction is less instructional than adult–child interaction, it still carries the potential to affect children's cognitive development.

THE SOCIAL CONTEXT OF PROBLEM-SOLVING INTERACTION

Recognition of the social nature of children's problem solving does not mean that this process proceeds in the same way for all children or all dyads. Characteristics of the child, the adult, the dyad, or the task may influence the course of joint problem solving, and these, in turn, may affect what children learn from social experience. The research used below to illustrate this point is not an exhaustive list of all the social–contextual factors that may contribute to this social–cognitive process. In fact, it is not clear that an exhaustive list is possible or worthwhile to generate. What is important is recognition of the complex interleaving of social and cognitive dimensions that compose thinking in social context. This, in turn, can help direct researchers' attention to these factors in their research. Over time, this may lead to a principled understanding of how the social context of cognitive experience relates to children's learning and development.

Characteristics of the Child

Many factors characteristic of the child may influence cognitive interaction. These include child age, individual cognitive skill, social competence, and emotionality. One or all of these may influence how cognitive interaction proceeds.

The question of whether children of different ages respond differently to adult assistance was taken up by Plumert and Nichols-Whitehead (1996) in a study examining children's spatial communication. This research concentrated on young children's ability to describe a spatial location in an unambiguous way—an important developmental achievement. Three- and 4-year-old children gave directions to parents about the location of a miniature toy mouse in a dollhouse. Parents were asked to respond to their children's directions by either asking for more explicit information about the location, a condition that was referred to as "direct prompts" (e.g., "Is it in the bag behind the TV?"), or by using more open-ended questions, called "nondirect prompts" (e.g., "Which bag do you mean?"), or by not questioning the child further. The researchers found age-related differences in how children benefited from these different forms of scaffolding, with 3-year-olds benefiting less than 4-year-olds from nondirect prompts. This suggests that there are important maturational contributions in early childhood, some that can emerge even in a 1-year period, that affect children's ability to benefit from social interaction with adults. Much of the research on scaffolding emphasizes the adult's contribution to the process. This study serves as a reminder of the importance of studying the children's contribution.

As another example of the role of child characteristics in social–cognitive activity, consider how child temperament, a measure of emotional adaptability and reactivity, may mediate parent–child joint problem solving. In a study involving 2½-year-old children and their mothers, children rated by their mothers as having more difficult temperaments when the children were 18 months old received more cognitive assistance and disapproval from their mothers during joint problem solving than children rated as having less difficult temperaments (Gauvain & Fagot, 1995). Mothers of children rated as temperamentally difficult assumed more responsibility for the more challenging aspects of the tasks, such as selecting which puzzle piece to insert next, than mothers of children rated as having an easier temperament (see Table 6.2). Although performance on the individual posttest was not directly related to child temperament, children who had more involvement in the more challenging aspects of the tasks during the interaction had better posttest performance. Such experience was more

TABLE 6.2. Means for Maternal Guidance, Mothers' and Children's Involvement in the More and Less Challenging Aspects of the Tasks, and Task Performance and Their Correlation with Child Temperament

Variable	Mean (SD)	Correlation with temperament rating
Maternal guidance		
Cognitive assistance	32.33 (14.4)	.38**
Behavioral directives	28.35 (15.6)	.33*
Positive support	19.61 (12.6)	.24
Disapproval	17.54 (10.1)	.38**
Mother's task involvement[a]		
More challenging aspects	2.45 (0.4)	.40**
Less challenging aspects	1.23 (0.3)	.12
Children's task involvement[a]		
More challenging aspects	2.49 (0.4)	.17
Less challenging aspects	2.95 (0.1)	.08
Task performance		
Interaction	15.35 (1.6)	.04
Posttest	7.08 (4.2)	.11

Note. From Gauvain and Fagot (1995). Copyright 1995 by Blackwell Publishers. Reprinted by permission.

[a] Average rating, using a 3-point scale (1 = never, 2 = sometimes, 3 = always) for each partner's active involvement in the more or less challenging aspects of the task.

$*p < .10$; $**p < .05$.

common among children rated as having an easier temperament. Apparently, children perceived by their mothers as easier or less difficult have more opportunity during joint activity to discover new strategies or to practice more complex actions under their mother's tutelage than children perceived by their mothers as more difficult.

These observations raise the question as to what information is used by adults during joint activity to help them regulate problem-solving interactions with their children. Usually in studies examining adult–child interaction, the assumption is that behaviors that arise during the interaction determine the guidance adults provide. However, research by Gauvain and Fagot (1995) discussed above suggests that other factors, such as parents' awareness of and sensitivity to their children's emotionality, may influence this process. Joint cognitive tasks may be especially likely to evoke parental sensitivity to children's temperament in that such tasks may exacerbate the behavior of children with difficult temperaments and thereby create a different learning context than that which occurs for dyads that include children who are perceived as having an easier temperament. These interpersonal experiences may leave traces later on in the child's development.

In a follow-up study involving these same children, both the mother's early perception of the child's temperament and her guidance during joint problem solving when the child was 2½ years of age were related to the child's problem-solving behavior at age 5 (Fagot & Gauvain, 1997). It is not possible to determine if the relations among the earlier maternal variables (child temperament rating, cognitive assistance) and the later child variables (child independent cognitive performance on two problem-solving tasks and class behavior as rated by the teacher) were due to initial differences in the child's abilities or whether the cumulative effects of parent–child interaction led to observed child behaviors at age 5. It is likely that both contributed to the patterns observed.

Characteristics of the Partner

Characteristics of the partner, whether an adult or a child, may also influence cognitive interaction. These include the relationship between the child and the partner, such as whether the adult is the child's parent or the peer is the child's friend. The expertise of the partner also matters, as I discussed above. Another important characteristic is the gender of the partner. Researchers who study the contribution of gender to joint cognitive activity have been especially interested in whether the cognitive guidance provided by mothers and fathers is similar or different.

In general, research that has compared the cognitive interactions of mothers and fathers with their children has found few differences in the behavior of mothers and fathers. Mothers and fathers are equally capable of identifying and using the child's region of sensitivity or zone of proximal development when instructing preschoolers (Conner, Knight, & Cross, 1997; Pratt, Kerig, Cowan, & Cowan, 1988) and school-age children (Gauvain, Fagot, Leve, & Kavanagh, 2000; Radziszewska & Rogoff, 1988, 1991). For example, Conner and colleagues (1997) observed 2-year-old children interacting with their mothers and fathers separately on two different occasions and on two different tasks. After the interactions, children worked on similar tasks on their own. One task involved problem solving (building a tower of blocks) and the other involved reading a book and having the child retell the story. Mothers' and fathers' behaviors were very similar during the problem-solving task. Both provided high levels of cognitive assistance and both were likely to shift their level of assistance appropriately when needed. Parental assistance during the interaction was related to the child's later individual performance, with more contingent, sensitive assistance by the parent related to better individual performance by the child on the posttest. This is the same type of pattern reported by

Wood and colleagues (Wood et al., 1976, 1978; Wood & Middleton, 1975) in their research. A different pattern of results appeared for the reading task, however. Mothers' behaviors were more contingently related to the child's behaviors than were the fathers' behaviors during joint reading.

A study involving parents and children in middle childhood reported similar task-related results, but it added child gender to the picture. Parental assistance for their 6-year-old children on two cognitive tasks, a puzzle and a picture memory task, was observed (Frankel & Rollins, 1983). Fathers provided more feedback, positive and negative, on the puzzle task, and mothers provided more feedback, positive and negative, during the memory task. Child sex was influential in that both parents were more performance- and task-oriented with sons and more cooperative with daughters, regardless of task.

Although both parents show differences across tasks, some research suggests that fathers are more affected by task than mothers. Worden, Kee, and Ingle (1987) found that mothers were more consistent than fathers in terms of verbal style on two tasks: reading picture books and interacting with alphabet-learning software on a computer. Worden et al. speculated that fathers' inconsistency across tasks may lead to increased difficulties for children when interacting with them relative to mothers. Other research supports this claim in that children appear to experience more communicative breakdowns with fathers than with mothers (Laasko, 1995; Tomasello, Conti-Ramsden, & Ewert, 1990). Fathers seem less skilled than mothers at adjusting their communication to the child's level. This may reflect the differential experience of mothers versus fathers in playing and working on joint cognitive tasks with their children (Parke, 1996). To summarize the data on mothers' and fathers' contributions to cognitive interaction with their children, it appears that both mothers and fathers are able to provide support for their children's learning during joint cognitive activity (Gauvain et al., 2000). The differences between mothers and fathers are relatively small given the large number of behaviors that have been examined and, in most cases, the differences observed were task-related.

Other characteristics of the partner have also been studied in relation to joint problem solving. For instance, parenting style appears to influence parent–child cognitive interaction. Pratt and colleagues (1988) found the authoritative parenting style positively related to more effective use by the parent of the child's region of sensitivity in joint problem solving. This suggests some link between parenting style and scaffolding when parents interact with their children. More personal qualities of the partner also appear to influence the nature of cognitive interaction. This includes factors like an individual's skill at teaching or working with young children (Rogoff & Gauvain, 1986). The partners' emotional state, such as whether he or she is depressed (Goldsmith & Rogoff, 1995) or has attention or compliance difficulties (Gauvain & DeMent, 1991), may also influence social interaction during joint problem solving. Essentially, child or adult behaviors that interfere with the sustained concentration, coordination, and support needed to make joint problem solving successful are likely candidates for influencing the nature of cognitive interaction.

Characteristics of the Dyad

Characteristics of the dyad may also lead to variation in social interaction during joint problem solving. Such characteristics may influence two aspects of the process. First, they may determine how the partners arrange the interaction. Second, they may influence the expectations partners have for each other's behavior during the interaction, which may, in turn, regulate one or both partner's participation during problem solving. In peer collaboration, many factors play a role. Several were discussed above, including the developmental status, relative expertise, and personal relationship of the partners. In parent–child interaction, dyadic characteristics like attachment and other descriptions of the dyad's shared social history are important to consider.

Patterns of mother–child problem solving have been found to be related to attachment classifications that were determined several months prior to a problem-solving interaction (Matas, Arend, & Sroufe, 1978). In this research, secure attachment was associated with more cognitive assistance and support by mother, as well as less off-task time, nay-saying, and aggression by children. Others have observed that mothers of insecure-avoidant and insecure-resistant babies provide a poorer quality of cognitive assistance during joint problem solving (Frankel & Bates, 1990). In other research, mothers of resistant children provided less task support and were more intrusive and disapproving during joint problem solving than mothers of children classified as securely attached (Fagot, Gauvain, & Kavanagh, 1996).

One study found that mothers and children in secure and insecure groups did not differ in terms of their general problem-solving approach, that is, the information they exchanged was comparable (Moss, 1992). However, in this research the affective tone of the interaction differed, with more mutual attention and coordination in the secure group. In the insecure group, the mutual attention that did occur was usually disapproving. The researchers also found that insecure children were less likely than secure children to comply with their mother's attempts to orient the child's attention to the task. This suggests that some sort of cycle of negative reciprocity may occur in insecurely attached dyads during joint cognitive activity. Moss also observed that mothers of insecure children did not scaffold children in the direction of behaviors that were developmentally appropriate, that is, in line with skills that were soon to appear. Rather, the mothers emphasized behavioral control, which discourages mastery and may interfere with the development of higher level strategies (Sigel, 1970).

CONCLUDING THOUGHTS

The main questions developmentalists ask about joint problem solving are whether cognitive development can benefit from these interactions, what roles different partners play over the course of these interactions, and whether task features or characteristics of either one or both of the partners are more likely to lead to positive cognitive outcomes. The past 20 years has seen a steep increase in studies examining how adult–child and child–child interactions relate to the development of problem-solving skills. The thesis at the center of these studies is the idea that experience with others leads to increased skill for children at solving problems. In order to evaluate whether these experiences contribute to the development of problem-solving skills, the benefits should be evident in how children encode problems, the strategies they use, and the knowledge base they draw on during problem solving.

Research on adult–child and child–child interaction suggests that solving problems with others may contribute to the development of children's problem-solving skills in each of these areas of growth. Children learn about encoding—specifically, what features of a problem space to encode—by observing more experienced partners (both adults and other children) solve problems. Whether these social experiences build on children's existing encoding skills, which is likely, or contribute to the formulation of encoding skills, is unknown. To date, evidence clearly supports the former conclusion, namely, that social experience can contribute to the refinement and more effective use of encoding skills. Although data do not currently exist to support the claim that solving problems with more experienced partners contributes to the formulation of encoding skills, this remains an open question.

Evidence that social experience can effect the development and use of strategies is substantial. The picture that is emerging is complex, however. Essentially, strategy use during joint problem solving is related to a greater likelihood that children will use these same strategies during later individual problem solving on related tasks. The type of evidence needed to support this point conclusively, namely, precise assessment of whether these strategies were in place before the joint activity occurred, is unfortunately still rare in research (Ellis et al., 1993). However, when such assessments have been conducted, evidence is mounting that children's use of strategies is affected by experience solving problems with others (see, e.g., Ellis, 1995).

Research examining strategy development and use has also asked whether scaffolding must be face to face or whether other forms of instruction are equally effective. This has been studied by providing children with problem-solving assistance on computers and by planting feedback on children's worksheets. The information provided to children during these "nonsocial interactions" aided their understanding and related to improved performance. However, it is important to emphasize that these types of nonsocial support were designed and staged by other people and not by the material artifact that conveyed the message. Like Piaget's experiments on knot tying described at the beginning of this chapter, the contribution of the social world is inherent even in these seemingly nonsocial performances. How these various types of social experiences can be mapped into a understanding of cognitive development in social context is on the agenda for the next decade of research on children's problem solving.

The third component of problem solving is the knowledge base. Clearly, joint problem solving enhances children's knowledge, especially when children interact with more experienced partners, either adult or child. The knowledge conveyed in joint activity is mostly domain-specific, and most of the research evidence described above illustrates this contribution to development. Adults are also active in children's early years in building conceptual structures that may be less tied to specific domains but help construct the foundation of knowledge that is used later in problem solving—for example, by pointing out to children that objects can belong to a group of objects with similar properties.

Cultural knowledge is also implicit in joint problem solving, most notably with adults, but this can also occur in child–child interaction. As Goodnow (1990) states, "The social environment does not take a neutral view toward the acquisition of knowledge and skill" (p. 260). When people solve problems together they convey lots of information in addition to task descriptions, procedures, and strategies. They also transmit a set of values about thinking in a particular domain in a particular cultural context. For example, adults may communicate information to children about the types of problems that are considered worth solving ("It is important for you to know this") and that some procedures are more valued than others ("This is the best way to do this"). In social context, children also learn about the categories of thinking that problems represent ("This is a math problem"), what solving a particular type of problem entails intellectually or emotionally ("Ooh, this is going to be hard to figure out"), and whether some problems are more suited to some individuals than others ("This is the kind of problem that mathematicians do"). Goodnow (1990) laments that there is far too little understood about this type of knowledge, how it is conveyed, and what difference it makes to children's learning. In her view, studying this will lead to a broader conception of what cognitive development is all about.

The next chapter continues this discussion by focusing on the development of one particular type of problem-solving skill: planning. We live our lives in good part in the future, and skills that support our passage there—like anticipating and determining future behaviors—are critical to social, cognitive, and emotional development.

Chapter 7

Constructing the Future: Planning in Social Context

*T*he Incan Empire existed from about c. 1200 to 1560. This civilization covered a vast area of South America, encompassing all of the land that is now Peru, along with parts of Ecuador, Bolivia, Chile, and Argentina. One of the remarkable features of the Incan civilization is that it did not have a written language. How, then, was it able to develop, coordinate, and maintain an extensive agricultural, mining, religious, and political system until destroyed by the Spanish in the late 16th century?

In order to function as a civilization, the Inca needed to have some regular and efficient form of communication throughout the region. Among the Incan artifacts that have been discovered, a particular artifact called a *quipu* has been found (Ascher & Ascher, 1981). A quipu is a collection of cords, typically made of cotton, with knots tied in it (see Figure 7.1). Quipus were used to record and communicate information about different aspects of the community, such as census figures, tax schedules, the output of gold mines, and the contents of food stores. They also may have contained the myths and oral history of the culture. Quipus were rather small in size, usually weighing less than a pound. Therefore, they were easy to bundle up and transport. Quipus were carried throughout the empire by a succession of runners on the extensive Incan road system. What were these messages like?

The basic units of the quipu were the individually constructed cords, which were composed of knots. Depending on how the cords were dyed, how they were connected to one another, how they were

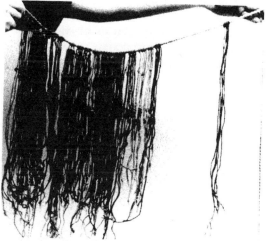

FIGURE 7.1. A photograph of a quipu that has been completed in unrolled form. Reprinted from Ascher and Ascher (1977, p. 33, plate 2.5). In the collection of the Smithsonian National Museum, Washington, DC. Photo by Marcia and Robert Ascher. Reprinted by permission.

spaced, the type of knots that were used, and the placement of the knots, different logical–numerical recording was possible. Only three types of knots were used: single knots (simple overhand knots), long knots (made up of two or more turns), and figure-eight knots. In order to use the knots to communicate a logical or mathematical value, the knot type and arrangement needed to be planned very carefully. As Ascher and Ascher (1981) explain:

> Depending on what is to be recorded, the assigning of numbers as labels and the assembling of numbers that express magnitudes are part of the planning of the quipu. The sizes of numbers have to be considered in order to select the length of the cords to be used . . . the maximum number of clusters on any cord of a particular quipu determines the placement of the clusters on other cords of the quipu. After deciding on the placement of the knot clusters, the knots must finally be tied in the cords of the prepared blank quipu. From the partially completed quipus, it is evident that the cords were not necessarily knotted serially from one end of the quipu to the other. (pp. 32–33)

Careful planning went into making each quipu so that the information it contained was clear and accurate. What resulted was a highly portable, decipherable code that allowed the Inca people to share with one another, over a vast land area, knowledge that was important to the group. Cultural artifacts like quipus provide us with a glimpse at commonalties in human intellectual activity over time and in different cultural circumstances. In this case, quipus illustrate the important role that planning has in individual cognitive activity and in social and cultural life. The unique use of knots in the quipu is especially intriguing. Here we see the adaptation of a simple, ubiquitous human behavior in the service of complex planful action that helped unite a social community.

In this chapter, I address the cognitive process of planning. I discuss what planning is, why it is important, and how children learn about planning from others. Just as apprentice quipu makers needed to learn from more experienced individuals how to plan out the arrangement of cords and knots, children throughout the world learn much about planning from those around them. The research I describe below examines how planning changes over childhood, with particular attention to the role of social experience in the organization and development of this important intellectual skill. Some of this research describes the different ways in which future-oriented concerns are woven into children's everyday lives, even from the very first year. Other research uses laboratory techniques to investigate how experience planning with adults or other children may contribute to the development of planning in specific ways. In addition to describing age-related changes in planning in social context, I highlight general themes that explain how the social process that emerges during an interaction may influence or regulate the development of planning in social context. I begin with a definition of planning and a brief account of the development of this skill when children plan on their own. This information serves as a backdrop for examining the social contributions to this developmental process.

PLANNING AND ITS DEVELOPMENT OVER CHILDHOOD

Planning is the deliberate organization of a sequence of actions oriented toward achieving a goal. It occurs both before and during action and is adapted to the circumstances of an activity (Rogoff, Gauvain, & Gardner, 1987). Planning is a complex cognitive skill that draws on a wide range of intellectual capabilities, including perception, attention, memory, and content knowledge. Planning is central to mature cognitive and social functioning. In fact, a basic assumption of human development is that with age children will have greater regulation of their own activities, a process that relies in critical ways on the ability to plan (Kopp, 1997). Planning skills help children carry out complex actions when they work on their own. These skills also help children coordinate actions with others—an experience that increases in frequency and importance over the years of childhood.

Like problem solving, planning involves a goal, means to reach the goal, and one or more obstacles that interfere with reaching the goal. So what distinguishes planning from problem solving? Although these processes are intertwined in many ways, they can be distinguished on a few grounds. The primary difference is that planning involves the anticipation and delineation of future-oriented actions, whereas problem solving is integrated with action in the here-and-now. Thus, planning relies more on metacognitive understanding than problem solving does. This is evident when you think about what makes someone good at either of these skills. Whereas good problem solvers are able to carry out goal-directed actions, good planners are knowledgeable about what they hope to accomplish, aware of the steps and strategies that may lead to that goal, and understand how to allocate attention to the various aspects of a situation. It is important to point out, as the last itemized skill implies, that planning sometimes occurs during action, that is, during problem solving. In such cases the distinction between planning and problem solving is muddied. For heuristic purposes, my discussion depicts a sharper distinction between these two cognitive processes than exists in the actual flow of behavior. I have done this in order to emphasize the unique contributions that social interaction has to each of these important cognitive processes.

Opportunities to plan with others can help children learn how to devise future-oriented actions, especially how to identify, evaluate, and select from alternative actions or strategies those that may be useful for reaching a goal. In terms of their developmental trajectories, planning skills emerge later than problem-solving skills, though, as we shall see, even infants possess a rudimentary ability to engage in planning-related processes. Planning skills emerge later in development than problem-solving skills for a number of reasons. For one thing, planning includes components, like anticipation, that are not present in problem solving (Das, Kar, & Parrila, 1996). Thus, planning is more cognitively demanding. In addition, certain cognitive abilities essential to planning, like the ability to represent action sequences and to manipulate them mentally in relation to particular outcomes or goals, emerge gradually over childhood. Because of these differences, problem solving and planning are involved in and benefit differently from social experience during the years of childhood. In particular, the cognitive demands of planning often leave children, especially young children, reliant on adults when they want to do activities that involve future-oriented action. Collaboration during planning is also affected by age-related changes in language and communicative competence, as well as by social skills

Before we examine the social contributions to the development of planning, a brief review of what we know about how children plan on their own over the course of childhood is in order.

The Development of Planning When Children Plan on Their Own

With development children become increasingly competent at planning in advance and during action, at allocating cognitive resources to various planning demands, and at mastering other metacognitive skills and strategies important for planning, such as organizing task materials and remembering the steps of a plan (Friedman, Scholnick, & Cocking, 1987; Haith, Benson, Roberts, & Pennington, 1994). Researchers have studied planning in children as early as the first year. They have observed such planning-related actions of infants as the ability to bypass a barrier to retrieve an object (Willatts, 1990), visual anticipation of a forthcoming event (Haith, 1994; Reznick, 1994), and control over motoric actions, like reaching or crawling (Benson & Haith, 1995; von Hofsten, 1994). These observations suggest that infants possess some rudimentary form of planning as early as 9 months of age. However, these actions are probably better described as future-oriented or planning-related behaviors rather than as planning per se. The former description is more appropriate because they do not unequivocally involve the representational skills and control over action alternatives that are essential for "true planning behavior" (Haith, 1997). However, as Haith suggests, it is likely that these behaviors indicate an emerging understanding of the future that is foundational to the development of planning.

Beyond the first years, planning skills develop gradually. Preschoolers can devise and execute simple plans in advance of action—for example, searching for a set of items in a play area (Wellman, Fabricius, & Sophian, 1985). They are also able to use knowledge of familiar events to plan a series of errands in a play store (Hudson & Fivush, 1991), and they are capable of solving problems that involve up to two moves on a simplified version of the Tower of Hanoi (Klahr & Robinson, 1981). The Tower of Hanoi is a problem that involves rearranging a stack of rings or disks across a set of pegs by moving only one ring or disk at a time and by following certain rules regarding the movements, such as a larger ring can never be positioned on top of a smaller ring. By 5 years of age, children have a fairly good conceptual understanding of what planning is and when it is needed (Pea, 1982), they are able to solve problems that require arranging four to five moves in advance (Klahr & Robinson, 1981), and they consider more alternatives and correct planning errors more readily than preschoolers (Fabricius, 1988). In middle childhood, children participate in increasingly complex activities, many of which rely on the ability to plan. For example, over the school years children show increasing competence at devising effective plans for accomplishing a set of chores (Pea & Hawkins, 1987) and for studying a text to prepare for an examination (Brown & Campione, 1984).

In sum, the development of competence at planning is a lengthy process. Children are able to reach adult levels of performance on certain tasks, such as errand planning, by middle childhood. But on more complex tasks, like those requiring complex computation or interpretation, adult-level performance is not reached until adolescence or later (Krietler & Krietler, 1987; Parrila, Aysto, & Das, 1994; Presson, 1987).

What accounts for these age-related developments in planning? Explanations for these changes are twofold. First, with development children are better able to regulate and suspend voluntary action, which permits greater opportunity for mental consideration of alternative procedures prior to action (Luria, 1976; Vygotsky, 1981). This capability may be related to maturational changes in the frontal lobe, which is centrally involved in consciousness and the regulation of activity (Fuster, 1989; Goldman-Rakic, 1987; Johnson, 1997; Pribram & Luria, 1973). A second explanation stresses the role of experience in the development of planning. The underlying assumption here is that with experience children come to understand the various components, benefits, and trade-offs of planning and, as a result, demonstrate increased incorporation of these skills in their activities.

As in all areas of development, both biological and experiential contributions are complementary processes that build upon and advance one another. In this chapter I concentrate on the experiential side of this relation, addressing how one particular type of experience, social experience, contributes to the development of planning skills in childhood. Because the social world is central to children's everyday experience, researchers are interested in knowing whether and what kind of experience with other people may provide children with important information about and practice with planning.

SOCIAL INTERACTION AND THE DEVELOPMENT OF PLANNING

Much of everyday planning, especially for young children, occurs in social settings as other people elicit and model planning-related behaviors for children. Such experiences may provide a formative base for the development of planning skills; research tends to support this claim. Children learn about planning as they coordinate plans with others and as they observe and interact with others who are more experienced planners (Gauvain, 1992; Gauvain & Rogoff, 1989; Radziszewska & Rogoff, 1988). Research has examined children's planning with adults and with other children, and has showed in both cases that these experiences may lead to the development of planning skills. Because of the different roles that adults and other children play in children's lives, and because of the different competencies that adults and children bring to joint cognitive activity, experience planning with adults versus planning with children contribute in different ways to the development of children's planning.

Planning with Adults

Future-Oriented Experiences in Infancy and Toddlerhood

There is little research on the role of adults in supporting the development of planning when children are very young. However, two related lines of research, both examining the interactions of parents and children, provide interesting insights. One area examines how adults discuss behavioral intentions with young children. The second area examines if and how adults talk to young children about the future. Both understanding of intentionality and knowledge of future events are clearly related to planning, and they may be stepping-stones in the development of this skill. Research on these topics suggest that social interaction, even at the very beginning of the child's life, may help set the stage for the development of understanding that appears fundamental to planning.

Intentionality. Even before infants begin to speak, adults talk to them about what they intend to do. For example, before getting a baby dressed to go out, a mother may ask the baby if she wants to go on a little trip. Or as a mother ties a bib around her baby's neck she may ask him if he wants to eat. These examples, which are emblematic of much of routine caregiving, illustrate how parent–child interaction often involves communication about the future.

It is important to remember that parents are not the only ones involved in these transactions. Infants are active participants from very early on. The basic communicative skills that infants need to participate in these interactions appear around 2 months of age. At this time infants start to respond to parental overtures by making sounds similar in pitch to the parent's voice (Snow, 1990). Gestures about intentions also play a role in these early "conversations." When infants are 7 to 8 months of age, adults begin to use pointing to direct infants' attention to events or objects of interest (Adamson, 1995). The use of simplified speech forms, or "motherese," to talk to babies facilitates the infant's engagement in these early social interactions (Newport, Gleitman, & Gleitman, 1977). Many of these behaviors, both verbal and nonverbal, are efforts to draw the infant's attention to future events. A parent's pointing often indicates to the baby where to look next, and the baby's active interest propels these interactions along. Verbal comments may describe forthcoming events. The following example of a mother's *extension*, a grammatically correct and enriched version of the child's ungrammatical statement, illustrates this interaction:

CHILD: (*pointing to dog*) Doggie.

MOTHER: Yes, there's a doggie.

CHILD: Doggie go.

MOTHER: Yes, the doggie is going away.

In this interaction, both mother and child direct their attention to a future action, and the extension provided by the mother reiterates and elaborates on this fact.

Much of social interaction, especially between adults and young children, refers to explicit behavioral intentions or goal states, and sometimes includes a means for achieving the goal. For Bruner (1982), this is inherent in the socialization process, which is designed to shape "human action into a highly intentional form" (p. 35). This is illustrated in the following comments made by mothers to their children who were early in the second year (Greenfield, 1980). One mother asked her son, "You wanna play patty-cake with Mommy?," and another asked her daughter, "Do ya wanna comb the baby's [referring to a doll] hair?" Intention–action statements such as these are used by adults to encourage the child to engage in a future action, either with the adult (play patty-cake) or alone (comb the doll's hair). Interactions like these provide the child with experience that links present activity (in this case, conversation) with future action—which is a prerequisite form of understanding that is essential to planning.

Once children begin to speak, much of their communication, especially to parents, is designed to share their intentions or future goal states. In fact, because young children are reliant on adults to help them conduct many of their activities, such communication occurs frequently in adult–child interaction in the early years of childhood. Bruner (1982) observed 2-year-old Richard as he attempted to get his mother, who was sitting nearby, to help him reach a goal.

> RICHARD: Mummy, Mummy, Mummy, come . . . up, up, up . . . cup-
> board . . . up cupboard, up cupboard, up cupboard . . . get up . . .
> cupboard, cupboard . . . cupboard up, cupboard up, cupboard up,
> telephone . . . Mummy . . . Mummy get out telephone. (p. 33)

Richard clearly wants to get something out of the cupboard that is out of his reach and he is trying to get his mother to get it for him. Note that his speech contains a three-step action sequence: he wants his mother to get up, he wants her to go to the cupboard, and he wants her to get the telephone out of the cupboard. Presumably, a fourth, unspoken step is implied, that is, mother is to give the telephone to Richard. Young children and their parents regularly engage in planning-related transactions such as this. Early in the child's life, these are primarily introduced by adults, as Greenfield's examples illustrate. With development children assume a larger, very active role in these discussions, as in the example provided by Bruner.

What do discussions between parents and children about intentions have to do with the development of planning? These interchanges are clearly planning-related in that they bring together means and goals directed toward the future. They may provide children with opportunities to learn about future-oriented behaviors. However, in order to be effective in helping children learn, they need to occur more than once or twice. Do future-oriented transactions occur often enough for children to learn much about planning from them?

Future-oriented talk. Talk about the future is commonplace in family discussion from very early in children's lives—even before children have much conceptual grasp of events beyond the present. Parents of infants between 9 and 36 months of age report that they regularly talk to their children about the future (Benson, 1994). Much of this talk pertains to the routines and organization of the day, although sometimes it includes activities that are weeks or even months away (see Figure 7.2). Do parents think that their children understand what they are talking about when they talk about the future? Not really, but they do it anyway and consider it instructional for their children. Of course, as children get older, between 30 and 36 months of age, parents do believe that their children are beginning to understand events that will occur farther into the future than the same day. However, even when children reach this age, parents recognize that their understanding of the future is far from perfect. As a mother of a 36-month-old boy explained, "Sometimes he gets the words mixed up and I think the concepts too. He calls tomorrow 'tomoyo' and a lot of times it means today" (Benson, 1994, p. 387).

Observations of mothers talking with their 2-year-old children indi-

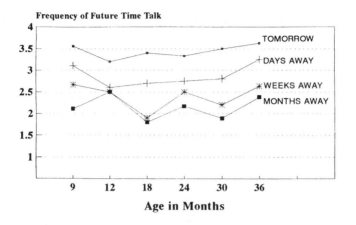

FIGURE 7.2. Age trends for mean ratings of future time talk (with 1 = rarely). From Benson (1994). Copyright 1994 by University of Chicago Press. Reprinted by permission.

cate that more than three-quarters of their conversations focused on future-oriented routines and events (Lucariello & Nelson, 1987). Children's contributions in these interactions included future-oriented references like the terms "later," "after," and "when." Does this mean that children of this age have a clear understanding of the future? A case study of a young girl named Emily helps answer this question (Nelson, 1989).

This study was conducted over a 16-month period, starting when Emily was 1 year and 9 months of age. It involved audiotape recordings of bedtime conversations between Emily and her parents, as well as Emily talking to herself after her parent(s) left her room and before she fell asleep. Over the course of the study, Emily's use of future-oriented terms, and presumably her understanding of these terms, changed (Levy & Nelson, 1994). Early in the observations her use of future-oriented terms mimicked the terms her parents used in their bedtime conversations with her—for example, "tomorrow morning" and "after a nap." Because Emily did not demonstrate flexible use of these terms, her understanding appears to have been quite limited at this time. Early in her second year, temporal reference terms almost entirely dropped out of Emily's self-talk. Then, shortly after turning 2½ years of age, she began to use future terms again. At this point the terms were no longer exact imitations of her parent's speech. Yet they were usually attached to activities and achievements—for example, "tomorrow when we wake up from bed." Thus, her use of temporal referents was showing some flexibility though they were tied to specific activities. It was almost as if each activity had a time slot, as in the statement "afternoon Daddy coming." This suggests that Emily's conceptual understanding of these terms was still developing at this point (Nelson, 1996). Even at age 3 Emily did not have the ability to interpret and construct temporal relations in an unrestricted fashion.

Emily's progress in using temporal referents reflects the pattern of understanding of the temporal and causal ordering of events that has been shown in other research with children of these same ages (Bauer & Mandler, 1990). It is not until late in the preschool years that flexibility in using temporal expressions in speech appears (Nelson, 1996). It is unknown just how much conceptual understanding of temporality and causal ordering is related to the development of planning, though presumably they have a central role. What is interesting is that, despite the conceptual and linguistic limitations in the first few years, much of adult–child interaction during this period involves future-oriented talk. Although no research directly links this type of talk to the development of planning, it is clear that concern with planning is woven into the regular family interaction process (Gauvain & Huard, 1999). As a sustained socialization context, parents and children regularly engage in conversations about what will happen next. Thus, by its nature, the family setting is a primary social context for the development of skills essential to an understanding of planning. Both parents and children, from early in the child's life, are active participants in these future-oriented discussions as they coordinate and direct future actions in ways that satisfy their mutual interests and needs. The early, frequent, and valued place these discussions occupy in communication between parents and children may provide a formative context for the development of children's planning.

Planning in Early and Middle Childhood

Between the ages of 4 and 11 years, children's skill at planning changes dramatically. Does planning with a more experienced partner contribute to the development of children's skill at planning during this time? Several studies have attempted to answer this question, and each sheds some light on how social experience may connect with these developing competencies.

In one study, 4- to 5- and 7- to 8-year-old children and their mothers were observed as they planned a series of errands using a tabletop model of a grocery store (Gauvain, 1992). Following the interaction, individual children took a posttest during which each child planned several shopping trips on his or her own. Two measures were used to describe planning on this task. One measure was verbally based and focused on the type of planning-related guidance or assistance the mothers provided for the children during the interaction. The other measure concentrated on nonverbal efforts that were planful in nature. Of particular interest was the extent to which the dyads (during the interaction) or the children (during the posttest) used visual search to locate the items before moving the toy shopper to fetch them.

Results revealed age-related differences in how mothers talk to children about planning. Mothers working with younger children concentrated on establishing joint understanding of the task with their children. They talked mostly about task structure, such as the rules and the organization of the task materials, and gave their children lots of feedback about their performance. In contrast, mothers who worked with older children emphasized strategy, that is, how to collect the items on the lists in a planful and systematic way. The two age groups also differed in their use of visual search strategies, with more visual search by dyads involving older than younger children. These patterns suggest that adult assistance during joint planning is tailored to developmentally related skills.

Did planning during the interaction relate to the children's later individual planning? In part it did. The use of visual search by dyads involving older children was related to more use of visual search by the older children when they planned later on their own. This relation did not appear for the younger children. Apparently older, but not younger, children were learning something by planning with an adult that was useful for the development of their own planning competence. There was no relation between mothers' discussion of strategy during the interaction and children's planning on the posttest. However, mothers' talk about task structure was negatively related to children's planning on the posttest. This finding is consistent with the view that more attention to task structure may indicate less understanding of the task on the part of the child. This pattern of results suggests that planning with an adult facilitates children's use of planning strategies later on when they plan alone. This only appeared for children in the years of middle childhood who may be more able to understand and adopt these strategies. For younger children, such strategies are less important because these children are still developing basic understanding of tasks that require planning.

These patterns are consistent with Vygotsky's (1978) notion of the zone of proximal development in that the more experienced partners, the mothers, involved the less experienced partners, the children, in the task in ways that were challenging for them. What was challenging for the children differed by age. The younger children, for whom the task was difficult, were given more opportunity to work on task structure accompanied by the adult. Their efforts to establish intersubjectivity concentrated on the structural features of the activity because this is what was challenging for them. Children who were more competent on the task, namely, the older children, received less structural guidance and feedback from the adult. For them the task was challenging in a different way. They received primarily strategic assistance from their adult partner, and this assistance benefited the children later when they planned alone. However, the benefits appeared in relation to the older children's participation in these strategies and not from the adults' discussions of strategy. It would be easy to see this social process as totally one-sided, that is, as controlled by the mother. But notice that none of the age-related adjustments could have been made by the mothers without active participation from the children. The children's behaviors informed the mothers about how to construct their assistance on this task; hence social co-construction occurred.

Before we conclude that exposure to talk about strategy plays no role in children's opportunities to learn about planning from social experience, we need to look at research on adult–child planning that involved children older than 8 years of age. What we see in this research is that the verbal requirements of planning may interfere with younger, but not older, children's learning about planning strategies from another person. Radziszewska and Rogoff (1988) compared adult–child and peer dyads that involved children between the ages of 9 and 11 years. The partners planned errands for several shopping trips using a map of an imaginary town, and then children planned another trip on their own. (Results from this study for adult–child planning are discussed here; the peer results are presented later in the chapter.) Children's posttest performance was related to their interactional experience in several ways. Children who planned with parents in dyads in which there was a high proportion of multiple-step plans, that is, sequences with two or more stops per planning step, and that included more extensive visual exploration of the map devised more efficient shopping routes when they planned later on their own. In addition, parents' verbal expression of strategies (a type of talk that rarely occurred in the peer dyads) was related to better posttest performance by the child. Finally, children who worked with adults who made strategy statements were observed using the behaviors discussed in these strategies in their individual planning. For example, one of the strategies that parents discussed, which was the optimal strategy for accomplishing this task, involved using colored pencils to mark the stores on the map that were included in a particular shopping trip. Children who worked with parents who discussed this strategy were more likely to use it later when planning alone than were children whose parents did not discuss this strategy.

Was there one best method for helping children learn to plan on this task? Closer analysis of the dyads in which children had the best posttest performance indicated that parents who helped children learn about planning behaved in a variety of ways. Some used a verbally didactic approach, that is, they described the strategy and posed good questions to the children. Other parents prompted their children to explore the task actively as the parents provided children with guided suggestions that were rich in strategy information. In comparison, in the less successful dyads, children often played a more instrumental role, that is, the parent told the child what to do or the parent dictated strategy steps one at a time until the task was completed (e.g., the parent would tell the child to mark all the stores and the child would comply, then the parent would tell the child to connect the marked stores with a line and the child would comply, etc.). Little verbal elaboration regarding the strategy being used accompanied this exchange.

This research tells us that exposure to talk about strategy is more likely to help children learn about planning as children get older. This not only reflects children's better planning skills, it also shows how changes in communicative competence contribute to what children learn in social context. It also suggests that different forms of social interaction may provide children with different opportunities to participate in and learn about planning. The more successful approaches differed in some ways, but they all involved active participation by the children. Less successful approaches relegated children to more passive roles.

Peer Planning

No research examines peer planning in the first years of life. However, there has been extensive study of peer planning in the early and middle years of childhood. A good deal of what has been learned about peer influences on children's planning comes from research in which peer planning has been compared with adult–child planning. The basic findings from these studies parallel those of similar research in the area of problem solving described in the previous chapter. Planning with an adult is related to better planning during joint activity than either planning with a peer or planning alone for children in early (Gauvain & Rogoff, 1989) and middle childhood (Radziszewska & Rogoff, 1988). When children and adults plan together they devise more efficient plans, and the adult's concern with strategy in particular is related to better individual performance by the child at a later time. Are there any unique contributions that peers make to this developmental process? To answer this question, we first need to examine what peers do when they plan together.

What Do Peers Do When They Plan Together?

When children plan with adult partners, especially older children, much of the adult's attention is focused on overall strategy. The adult tends to treat the planning problem as a single problem with multiple steps that need to be coordinated in order to reach the goal. In contrast, during joint planning among peers, the partners tend to focus on immediate planning steps. In other words, they treat the problem more like a set of isolated steps and less like an integrated problem composed of several moves. This orientation to the problem goes hand-in-hand with another propensity in peer planning: peers are quite concerned with coordinating their actions (Radziszewska & Rogoff, 1988), that is, deciding who gets to do what, whose turn is next, and so forth. The more children concentrate on these types of social behaviors when they plan together, the worse they do during joint planning and the less they learn about planning from the interactional experience. Thus, both behaviors, namely, less strategic concern and more attention to social coordination, are related to poorer performance overall. Again, the concomitant development of social, cognitive, and emotional competence collide, and the challenges presented by the development of certain skills, in this case strategy knowledge and social coordination, dominate children's activity.

Although concentration on immediate planning steps, essentially single-step planning, gets the task done, it ignores aspects of the overall planning space that are critical for solving the problem in an effective way. The reasons children do this when they plan together is unclear. Given the fact that by middle childhood children are able to work on multiple-step plans on their own, this pattern is puzzling. It may be that coordinating the social aspects of joint activity keeps children from formulating multiple-step plans that are clearly integrated with and directed toward the task goal. Negotiating roles and responsibilities is not easy for children. In many instances children resolve this either by dividing the task between them and then taking turns, or by one child dominating the activity and the other playing either an instrumental role or simply acting as an observer. Both of these types of social behaviors appear to interfere with learning about planning from collaborating with a peer relative to an adult.

Planning with an Adult versus Planning with a "Trained" Peer

Perhaps some of the limited understanding of planning strategies that is fostered by peer collaboration can be remedied if a peer is made knowledgeable of effective planning strategies on a task. However, research has shown that even when peers are trained to use the optimal planning strategies that adults use, collaboration with a peer still does not yield as good a planning outcome as collaboration with an adult (Radziszewska & Rogoff, 1991). Some noteworthy differences did occur in the trained/untrained peer comparison (see Table 7.1). When peers are trained to use the optimal strategy, the peer partners tend to use more elaborate, multistep plans, just like adult–child partners. This suggests that children, at least in the 9- to 11-year-old range, are able to use more sophisticated planning approaches when working with a peer, but that this is likely to occur only when this approach is pointed out to the child(ren) before collaboration begins. However, even when peer partners in this research used more sophisticated planning strategies, similar to those that adults use, their use was not, as is the case in adult–child planning, related to better planning on the later individual posttest. This may be explained by two characteristics that differentiated the adult–child and the trained-peer dyads. First, children were more actively involved in decision making when they worked with an adult than with a trained peer. This suggests that adults are more skilled at the social demands of collaboration, which then enhances children's opportunity to learn in this context. Second, even though adults and trained peers used the same optimal strategy to plan their errands, adults were more likely to verbalize this strategy in the partner's presence. They thereby provided instruction and explanation to the child about this approach to planning.

TABLE 7.1. Means (and Standard Deviations) of Joint Planning Process and Posttest Performance in Different Dyadic Conditions

	Dyads		
Process/performance	Untrained peer	Trained peer	Parent
One-step moves	$16.8^{a,b}$	3.2^{a}	3.0^{b}
	(7.2)	(3.3)	(4.3)
Average planning unit	$1.5^{c,d}$	3.5^{c}	4.5^{d}
	(0.9)	(1.6)	(2.4)
Collaborative route length	$135.4^{e,f}$	119.7^{e}	112.7^{f}
	(16.4)	(11.2)	(6.6)
Target child posttest	133.4^{g}	126.2^{h}	$118.5^{g,h}$
route length	(14.5)	(10.1)	(9.7)

Note. Route lengths are reported in blocks traveled in the model town. The minimum possible number of blocks was 104 summed over two collaborative trials, and 106 for two posttest trials. Means with the same superscripts differed significantly at $p = .05$. From Radziszewska and Rogoff (1991). Copyright 1991 by the American Psychological Association. Reprinted by permission.

Thus, even though children in early to middle childhood seem sufficiently skilled at planning to benefit from working together, some of the social aspects of planning with a peer may interfere with children learning about planning in this social context. Peers do not talk much about planning strategies, a process that benefits children's learning about planning in a social setting. Children are also less skilled at social coordination, which may interfere with their opportunity to learn about planning in a peer context because it restricts children's participation in decision making during planning. Moreover, we know from other research that shared decision making is related to children's learning about planning in social context (Gauvain & Rogoff, 1989).

Because planning is in many ways a process of decision making as individuals analyze a problem space and decide on particular paths of action to solve the problem, less access to a partner's thinking about the task and to the actual decision making involved are bound to interfere with learning about planning when people plan together. Thus, even though peers tend to watch one another during peer planning, and therefore have some opportunity to find out about their partner's thinking from these observations, this may be insufficient for learning due to the nature of planning itself. That is, much of what is deliberated in planning is not demonstrated in overt behaviors but exists in mental consideration of alternative moves. All of these factors—less verbalization, social difficulties, and limitations on learning from observation in this context—lead to less learning about planning in the peer context relative to adult–child planning. This is true even when children are in the years of middle childhood and are fairly competent at planning on their own.

Collaboration and Learning When Planning with a Peer

Are there any peer arrangements that may yield more opportunity for children to learn about planning from one another? Some research indicates that the way in which the task is structured may influence how peers interact and what learning may ensue. Glachen and Light (1982) observed 8- to 9-year-old children as they solved the Tower of Hanoi problem. In this study, the movable pieces were fitted with a handle on each end. When children worked in pairs they were told that they had to pick up the rings together using the handles. Before the peer dyads worked on this puzzle together, each child was individually pretested to assess his or her skill at this puzzle. Following the interaction the children were involved in an individual posttest.

Children's performance in the individual and joint sessions were examined for the number of moves they used to solve the problem. The researchers also identified the patterns of goal-directed moves the children made, which they referred to as *strategies*. Using these criteria, children were identified as either *strategists*, that is, those who used a specific pattern of moves to solve the problem; *nonstrategists*, that is, those who succeeded in solving the problem but did not use any regular pattern of moves or strategy; or *failures*, that is, those who did not solve the problem and did not use a strategy.

The effect of peer interaction was examined by comparing children's pretest and posttest performances. Several interesting results emerged. Children who were nonstrategists on the pretest improved on the posttest regardless of social condition. Thus, practice of any sort was useful for children who were able to do the task but who did not use any regular pattern of moves or strategy. Children who had failed on the pretest showed little improvement regardless of social condition. Practice, regardless of the "packaging," is not helpful to children who are not able to do the task. Finally, children identified as strategists improved more following peer interaction than when they planned alone. Why? Perhaps this was due to the fact that among the children identified as strategists various skill levels were represented. Maybe only the most skilled children in this group showed gains. However, a follow-up analysis showed that the results could not be explained by differential improvements in the skill groups. Thus, children who used strategies on the individual pretest, regardless of their initial ability, and then worked in dyads improved more than children of this same skill level who used strategies on the pretest but then worked alone.

Glachen and Light (1982) were also interested in knowing whether the rate of collaboration itself explained these results. In a second study using this same apparatus, they investigated whether peer interaction that required collaboration led to different outcomes than peer interaction in which collaboration was not required. Recall that in the earlier study children were directed to pick up the rings together, but they did not have to do so in order to complete the task. Again, only the children who used strategies on the pretest showed improvement following the interaction. However, this result only appeared for children in the condition in which collaboration was required. Dyads in this condition shared responsibility for deciding 75% of their moves, compared to 10% in dyads in which collaboration was not required. What were the children in this latter group doing the other 90% of the time?

When social coordination among children in the "collaboration not required" group was examined, planning tended to be dominated by one partner rather than divided equally. Dominance in peer groups is a well-known feature of peer social relations in play contexts (Blurton

Jones, 1972). Therefore, it is not surprising to see it emerge, and have consequences, in a peer learning context. These results suggest that in peer learning contexts, concerns about social dominance do not promote conditions beneficial for learning, such as shared responsibility for decision making. Dominance appears to interfere with the emergence of learning opportunities during peer planning because it impedes the type of verbal exchange that is useful for learning about planning from others. Dominant partners tend to direct the moves of the submissive partners rather than instruct or collaborate with them.

The extent to which peer partners share responsibility for the task is not the only factor that may interfere with children learning from peer planning. Other factors, like the relative age of the partners, a factor directly linked to peer dominance, may influence peer interaction on cognitive tasks.

Which Matters More in Peer Interaction—Age Or Expertise?

In most studies of peer interaction on cognitive tasks, individual differences in expertise are assumed to correspond to age differences (Ellis & Gauvain, 1992). Although this may be a reasonable assumption, expertise on particular tasks does not necessarily correlate with age, especially ages that are somewhat close developmentally—for example, 5- and 7-year-old children. Preassessments of children's ability on tasks independent of age are essential for establishing skill level and assigning children to dyads.

A related concern is the influence of differential age on peer involvement during interaction. Recall that Piaget cautioned that interaction with adults may be less effective than interaction with peers due to inherent restrictions imposed by differences in status between adults and children. This may be important to consider in peer interaction in which peers are of the same age versus different ages. Research in social development indicates quite clearly that child age is correlated with social status and dominance (Blurton Jones, 1972; Grusec & Lytton, 1988), and, as Glachen and Light (1982) showed, dominance may not lead to beneficial social–cognitive interaction. This suggests that in peer collaboration age-related status may play an important role in determining how partners participate in the interaction. However, since age and expertise, even when preassessed, are typically confounded in developmental research, it is unclear how age-related status may affect peer interaction.

To explore this issue, Duran and Gauvain (1993) studied the role of age versus expertise in influencing collaboration during joint planning. Five- and 7-year-old children were identified on an individual pretest as either novices or experts on a planning task. The task was a route-scheduling task that involved sequencing and delivering a group of items to locations in a model town drawn on poster board. Five-year-old children identified as novices were paired with a 5-year-old or a 7-year-old identified as an expert. Following collaboration, the 5-year-old novices participated in an individual posttest on a similar version of the task.

Children's experiences during the interaction differed in these two peer groups (see Table 7.2). Novices who planned with same-age experts had more involvement in the task than novices who planned with older experts, and this involvement increased over the course of the interaction. Same-age experts provided their partners with more positive support during the interaction, although conflict between the partners was also somewhat greater in the same-age condition. This suggests that when children work with partners of the same age, even though expertise may differ, certain social behaviors, like support and challenge of another's point of view, are more likely to occur. These processes are related to learning. Involvement by the novice in the task was related to better posttest performance. Thus, as we saw in adult–child research, the extent to which novices are involved in a task influences learning. However, the extent of novice involvement is affected by the relative age of the social partners, and such involvement is more likely among same-age peers.

TABLE 7.2. Means for Percentage Involvement by Novices and Experts and for Frequency of Interactional Process by Group for the Interaction Tasks

Variable	Same-age dyads		Cross-age dyads	
	Delivery 1	Delivery 2	Delivery 1	Delivery 2
Partner's task involvement				
Novice only	28.6	34.6	29.8	22.9
Expert only	52.4	49.9	51.1	58.5
Both novice and expert	19.0	15.4	19.0	18.6
Guidance by an expert				
Physical intervention	1.4	3.2	1.4	1.6
Directives and suggestions	2.9	5.6	2.6	3.1
Positive support	1.6	5.1	1.5	1.2
Observational learning (in seconds)	22.0	50.0	19.0	18.4
Conflict	2.5	4.2	1.1	2.2

Note. From Duran and Gauvain (1993). Copyright 1993 by Academic Press. Reprinted by permission.

The reasons underlying this process are uncertain. Perhaps novices who planned with same-age experts did not perceive as much social and cognitive distance between them and the experts compared to novices who planned with older experts. Children may feel more comfortable collaborating with experts of the same age and may even perceive the partner's skills as attainable. Of course, another explanation may be that older experts dominated the interaction, which they did. So rather than the novice increasing participation across trials as the children became more familiar with the task, as was the case in the same-age pairs, 5-year-olds who planned with older experts showed decreased participation over the trials. This pattern, along with the fact that the 5-year-old experts provided more positive support for their partners, raises the possibility that the 5-year-old experts were more sensitive to the learners' needs and capabilities, and therefore allowed their novice partners to be more involved in the task as they gained experience. Of course, the related interpretation is that 5-year-old novices are more likely to allow older experts than same-age experts to dominate the interaction. A marginally significant difference in the amount of conflict in these two groups, which was higher in the same-age dyads, supports this interpretation. More frequent bids for dominance by older children and acceptance of these dominance bids by younger children are reciprocal processes, that, by definition, are more likely to appear in mixed-age pairs.

It is not known if these results generalize across different ages or if they are specific to the ages of children included here. Research on the development of social comparison processes (Feldman & Ruble, 1988; Ruble, Boggiano, Feldman, & Loebl, 1980; Ruble & Frey, 1987) indicates that child age is related to children's ability comparisons between themselves and others. During social interaction, 5- to 6-year-old children, that is, children the same age as the novices in the Duran and Gauvain (1993) study, are primarily oriented toward same-age peers as a source of social comparison. Older children and adults are more likely to select "upward" comparisons as a source for self-evaluation. Stated more generally, the meaning of different people in social–cognitive processes, like social comparison, is a function of age-related developmental processes. In this study, same-age experts may have constituted an ideal arrangement for mediating social–cognitive effects for 5- to 6-year-old novices, thereby reflecting age-specific processes of social comparison rather than more general principles of social facilitation across childhood.

In general, peer collaboration during planning leads to learning under certain conditions. Nevertheless, the influence of peers on the development of planning is less potent than that of adults. It should be noted that peers may contribute in other ways to the development of children's planning than research on collaborative tasks reveals. Peers may influence each others' planning in the context of social interaction that is designed to accomplish a social goal. Planning social behavior is more likely to occur in peer than in adult–child interactions because when children interact with adults, as research on adult–child interaction has shown, adults assume more of the responsibility for the social parts of the transaction.

Coordinating Social Behaviors with Peers: Planning Activities in a Social Setting

Learning how to plan and coordinate social behaviors is more likely to emerge during social experiences with peers than with adults. In fact, experience coordinating social life with age mates may be one of the unique contributions that peer interaction makes in the development of children's planning. Unlike planning with adults, which often includes *explicit* instruction or guidance, peer planning in social settings is largely an *implicit* process. This is because when social experiences are planned, partners rarely talk about the strategies they use or the goals they have. Therefore, it is reasonable to assume that children's opportunity to learn about social-planning processes from peers relies little on strategic discussions or explications of this process. Rather, children learn about social planning with peers primarily through their own attempts, their successes and their failures, and by watching the successful and failed attempts of other children.

As early as age 3, interacting with peers as children coordinate their future behaviors seems to lead to improvement in children's planning skills. However, at this point in development, children's self-concerns and their limited awareness of others' needs influence their coordination with others. Gearhart (1979) observed pairs of 3-year-olds as they arranged their play episodes in a pretend store. She found that children of this age were able to arrange some of their future play behaviors. Yet the children's plans lacked one ingredient that was essential for coordinating future play: they lacked consideration of the partner's perspective. In this game the children needed each other in order to play and so they tended to include their partner in their plans. However, the partner was not included as an independent agent who had plans of his or her own. Rather, the child tended to include the partner more like an instrument or tool in the accomplishment of the child's own plan. This involved telling the other child what to do and when. Interestingly, even at this young age, children learned that this approach did not work very well. Over the course of several planning episodes, they discovered that human beings do not serve as an effective tool in carrying out one's plans because they typically have plans of their own. Learning this lesson helped children coordinate plans more effectively during the later play sessions. In fact, during the later episodes children showed clear attempts to prearrange elements of social coordination that had caused them difficulty in earlier play episodes. This suggests that children as young as 3 years of age can learn something about planning through their own successful and failed attempts to plan or organize future behaviors with others.

Although children's learning about planning along these lines appears to be important, our understanding of how children engage in and learn about planning in social situations that involve peers is limited. This is because there are few studies, except Gearhart's research, in which children have been observed as they coordinate their own individual cognitive activities with the behaviors of others in everyday situations. To address this lack, Gauvain (1989) conducted an observational study of kindergartners' planning in the classroom. Children were observed on 10 occasions (once a week) during the 1-hour free-play period of the day, which was called "Free Choice." The first two observations established a baseline record of the children's activities during the period; they were followed by 7 weeks of observation in which children planned their activities for this period in advance, and ended with 1 week in which children were observed but did not plan in advance. Following the observations children were interviewed about their favorite activities and classmates (i.e., peer nominations).

During Free Choice, children were allowed to participate in any of 11 activities: art, blocks, chalkboard, climber, construction toys, housekeeping, library, listening (to tapes), puppets, sandbox, and table games. To study planning, these activities were listed on a plan recording sheet that was given to the children at the beginning of each day of observation. Figure 7.3 shows the planning sheet that children used in the planning sessions. Children were asked to list the activities they planned to do that day and the order in which they planned to do them. Children could plan as many activities as they wanted. Observations were conducted using a "scan sampling" technique (Altmann, 1974) in which children's activities were recorded at 5-minute intervals throughout the hour-long period.

What was children's planning in this complex, everyday, social situation like? Like adult planners (Hayes-Roth, 1980), children tended to overplan their activities. Although baseline observations showed that children did about three different activities during this period, children planned an average of six different activities during the 7-week observation period. Even though children planned an average of six activities,

My Name is _____

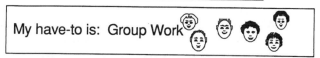

My want-to's are:

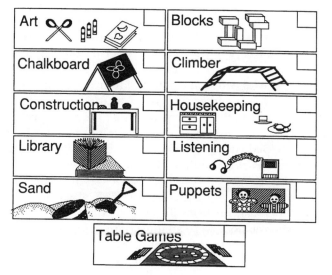

FIGURE 7.3. Example of the planning form completed by the children at the beginning of seven class sessions involving advance planning of Free Choice activities. From Gauvain (1989). Copyright 1989 by Ablex Publishing Corporation. Reprinted by permission.

they still actually did about three activities per 1-hour session. Interestingly, the number of activities children planned decreased over the observational sessions, from an average of 5.8 activities at the first session to an average of 4.6 activities at the last session, which is significantly different. This suggests that the children may have learned something about how much to plan for a 1-hour period from planning and executing their own ambitious and unrealized plans.

How similar were children's activities to their plans? Research involving children of this same age planning alone indicates that these children are good at carrying out one-step and two-steps plans. The kindergartners observed by Gauvain (1989) were most competent at planning and executing plans for the initial activity of the day. The correspondence between their plans and their actual activities dropped precipitously after the first activity. Some children were more successful than others at planning and executing more than one activity, however. Those who planned their favorite activities among the first three activities were more successful in carrying out their plans than those who tended to plan activities they did not identify as their favorites. Personal interest was apparently a motivating force for remembering and carrying out the plans. Was there any evidence that children were learning about the process of planning from this experience? Yes, there was, but what children were learning about planning was somewhat surprising. As early as the third planning session, children began to make overt efforts to revise their plans, either by altering them during the Free Choice period or by refusing to enumerate activities in advance. These behaviors indicate that children were monitoring their plans during execution and either trying to increase correspondence between their plans and their behavior or that they were trying to override the rigidity of the plans by not specifying the sequence. This latter strategy surely helped children maintain some flexibility while still planning. In other words, it helped the children meet both their own goals and the researcher's goals. For the researcher, the children's plans were about the activities. For the children, their plans were about both the activities and social relations in the classroom.

In fact, social relations were an important component of children's planning in this context. In the initial planning sessions, the plans devised by children rated as more popular by the other children in the class corresponded more with their behavior than those devised by the less popular children. However, the correspondence rate dropped swiftly for the popular children following the second advance planning session. Were popular children less effective planners? There is no evidence that indicates that this was the case. Rather, it seems that popular children wanted to play with their friends and this goal eclipsed the researcher's goal for the children to devise and keep to their plans. Interestingly, as the sessions wore on, all the children were increasingly likely to be at activities with children who they rated as their friends, regardless of what they planned. Why this behavior appeared earlier among the more popular children is an interesting question. Although more and less popular children are both concerned with social experience, popular children may be more willing or able to exercise control, when possible, over this experience. Less popular children may be more timid about exercising such control or they may have learned from observing the actions of their more popular classmates.

In sum, the 5-year-olds observed in this study displayed competence at making activity plans, monitoring their plans during execution, and following through on their plans, at least to some degree. When children did not follow through on their plans, this was explained by a number of factors including children's activity preferences and social relations in the classroom. Even though social relations appeared important, the children did not try to change the planning process in any way to accommodate this. Children did not try to discover their friend's plans before they made their own plans, nor did they try to coordinate their plans with those of their friends at the beginning of the day. This hints at a limitation young children may have as they plan in social settings. Although children of this age may be capable of modifying their plans when a social opportunity arises, they are not able to anticipate the importance or likelihood of these social opportunities in advance. These considerations involve anticipating several goals simultaneously. We know from other research that 5-year-olds have difficulty with this. The fact that the other children were also planning at the same time added complexity to the situation and may have made planning in this context particularly difficult for the children.

Coordinating Social Behavior with Peers: Planning Social Engagement

Research on children's planning with peers has also examined how children plan and execute social entry behaviors with other children during play. Forbes, Katz, Paul, and Lubin (1982) created an afterschool play group composed of 5- and 7-year-old children who did not know one another. The play group, which was recorded on videotape, met 12 times over a 3-week period in a laboratory playroom stocked with toys and games. A teacher was present, but in a side room, so the children's activity was not controlled by an adult. The researchers were interested in how children approached and initiated activity with children who were already at play, a process called *third-party entry*. To study this process, they coded all instances of third-party entry approaches, which they considered an example of social planning. Although both ages of children were equally successful in their third-party entry bids, the 7-year-olds used more sophisticated strategies to gain entry. They focused more on relational issues, such as asking if they could join the group. The 5-year-olds emphasized activity connections to the group, either by asking to join the activity or by proposing a new activity.

It appears that with increasing age children become more sensitive to the social aspects of group play, and this sensitivity influences how they plan social entry. Another piece of evidence in support of this interpretation is the fact that the younger, but not the older, children were more likely to use what the researchers called an "ignore and proceed" strategy. This occurred when the group gave the child who was bidding for entry negative feedback in order to discourage him or her from joining the group. Five-year-olds would proceed to join the group even when negative feedback was directed toward them, 7-year-olds would not.

The years from 5 to 7 are important in the development of many cognitive skills (Sameroff & Haith, 1996). The results of research by Gearhart (1979), Gauvain (1989), and Forbes and colleagues (1982) indicate that this may also be a critical time in the development of children's skill at planning and coordinating actions with peers in social context.

SOCIAL PROCESSES THAT REGULATE CHILDREN'S OPPORTUNITIES TO LEARN ABOUT PLANNING FROM EXPERIENCE WITH OTHERS

The following sections examine the social processes involved in planning interactions more closely. Research clearly indicates that some types of interactions are more likely than others to help children learn about planning in social context.

Script Knowledge and Children's Planning in Social Context

Some situations may be more conducive than others for young children to learn about planning when interacting with another person. One way to study this issue is to examine how children plan for a familiar event, such as grocery shopping. Young children's familiarity with an activity may mean they have a script for the activity, and the availability of a script may assist young children in learning about planning from others. This is because planning involves remembering a group of items of some sort. Script knowledge may lessen the memory load associated with planning because the items are already remembered in relation to the grouping contained in the script. This may be particularly helpful for young children for whom the multiple cognitive demands of planning may simply be too taxing.

We know from research that by 3 or 4 years of age children have a fair amount of experience shopping for groceries with their parents. In fact, by this age children often have a script for grocery shopping that includes the general structure of the activity and the overall arrangement of a grocery store and the items in it (Farrar & Goodman, 1992). When Hudson and Fivush (1991) examined the planning skills of young children while their planning was supported by script knowledge, they found that children could develop a plan as young as 3 years of age. The investigators then examined whether adult assistance during planning for a scripted event contributes anything to young children's planning beyond the support provided by the script. Note that two social contributions to planning are studied here. One is the use of a script, which is a social convention for organizing knowledge, to help children as they plan. The other is the assistance of a more experienced partner, the experimenter, in helping children plan their shopping for an event. Results pertaining to both of these forms of social support for the development of planning are discussed below.

Hudson and Fivush (1991) studied 3-, 4-, and 5-year-old children, who were observed as they planned and shopped for groceries for two familiar events, breakfast and a birthday party. The shopping was done in a small, simplified grocery store constructed in a laboratory. Two social conditions were observed. Some children planned and carried out the shopping on their own and some children planned and shopped with the help of a trained experimenter. In the latter condition, the experimenter provided the children with three types of information: feedback about the appropriateness of the items on the children's lists in relation to the events (e.g., "No, we don't usually eat spaghetti at breakfast"); suggestions for items appropriate to the event that were in the store but not on the child's list (e.g., "How about orange juice?"); and reminders during plan execution of the event ("Remember, you have to get everything for breakfast").

When 3-year-olds planned on their own, they were able to plan and shop successfully for one item at a time; this success was facilitated by script knowledge. When the item for which they were shopping was grouped with other like items on the shelves (e.g., a breakfast item was with other breakfast items), the 3-year-olds were more successful than when the items were not grouped together in this way. Assistance from the experimenter also helped the 3-year-olds plan on this task. With assistance, these children were more successful at creating one-item plans regardless of the location of the items, and some successful multiple-event (two-item) plans also occurred. Adult guidance had a different impact on 4-year-olds because of their different level of competence at the task. When these children planned alone they were able to shop for single items successfully regardless of shelf placement but they had difficulty shopping for two events simultaneously. When the adult helped them, they were able to do this with little difficulty. By 5 years of age, children were able to do the task successfully and external support, either from the contextual organization of the items in the store or adult assistance, added little to their performance.

This research reveals three important points about children's planning in the preschool years. First, young children are able to use knowledge about familiar events to construct plans. Second, social support in the form of reminders and evaluation can help young children when they plan for familiar events. Third, by age 5 children are able to plan short sequences of actions for a familiar event and adult assistance is not needed. This suggests that changes in competence as a result of social experience may be limited to the early stages of skill acquisition (Hawkins et al., 1984). These results do not indicate whether social experience can help 5-year-olds plan sequences of actions that are not linked to a scripted event. The following study addressed this question.

Gauvain and Rogoff (1989) observed 5-year-old children and their mothers as they planned several multiple-item shopping trips in a model grocery store. Items in each shopping list were not organized in relation to any scriptlike knowledge other than that they all could be found in a grocery store. Following the interaction, children planned several more shopping trips on their own. Children who planned with mothers who discussed the task rules and efficiency of the route being planned were more successful at planning shopping trips later on their own. Apparently, when 5-year-olds plan a route to retrieve lists of unrelated (i.e., nonscripted) items, adult assistance is helpful. This study also revealed information about an aspect of the social interactional process that may be particularly beneficial to children for learning from social experience. Talking about the task rules and strategies was useful in helping children learn about planning, but it was not sufficient. What also mattered was how much the dyad shared responsibility for decision making during the task.

Sharing Task Responsibility during Joint Planning

Gauvain and Rogoff (1989) found that children who worked in dyads that shared responsibility for locating the majority of the items were more planful in their actions and developed more effective plans on the posttest than children who worked in dyads that did not share as much responsibility for making decisions. Why does sharing responsibility matter? After all, didn't all the children have opportunity to observe the mother do the task?

Sharing responsibility aids children's learning in that it encourages joint task understanding or intersubjectivity (Rommetveit, 1985) during the interaction. This, in turn, may enhance children's understanding of the planning problem from the perspective of the more experienced partner. When dyads did not share much responsibility, the partners either took turns and did not help one another during each other's turns or the mother used the children instrumentally to carry out her plan ("OK, now get this one, it's over here"). Neither of these approaches were as helpful as including the child in decision making.

These results support Hartup's (1985) view that social interaction during a cognitive task may be related to the development of planning. The results extend this point by stressing that it is during interactions in which responsibility for decision making is shared that children are most likely to have opportunities to develop these skills. Although children may learn about problem solving by observing others (see, e.g., Azmitia, 1987; Bandura, 1977), sharing responsibility may be especially useful during tasks that involve planning. When actions are being planned, much of the cognitive activity occurs mentally. Because the benefit of one course of action versus another may not be visually apparent, being involved in decision making makes children privy to the planning considerations of the more experienced partner. For young children, in particular, joint involvement may be especially critical in helping them learn about planning from others.

These findings beg the question of whether adults usually share decision-making responsibility with children when they plan together. In the Gauvain and Rogoff (1989) study, fewer than half the mother–child dyads shared responsibility for more than half of the task. In fact, only three of the nine dyads shared responsibility for planning during most of the task. Why was the rate of sharing responsibility so low? Perhaps the children were too young to share much of the responsibility for deciding how to plan on this task. Or perhaps this pattern is explained by the way the activity was described to the participants at the outset. In this study, the task was presented as a game and not as an instructional situation—that is, the partners were not forewarned of the impending posttest for the child. In studies in which participants are aware of the child-only posttest, results consistently show active efforts by adults to involve the child partners and by children to learn about the task (see, e.g., Ellis & Rogoff, 1982; Radziezewska & Rogoff, 1988, 1991). In other words, the apparent goal of the activity may have influenced the way that the participants interacted, and this, in turn, may have affected what children learned from the social experience.

Influence of the Goal on How Adults and Children Plan Together

The idea that the goal of the activity influences behavior is consistent with a sociohistorical approach. In addition to the role that more experienced social partners may play in developing cognitive skill, another central premise of this approach is the idea that human behavior and thinking occur in meaningful contexts as people conduct purposeful, goal-directed action (Leont'ev, 1981; Wertsch, 1985). Different goals for joint activity may create different learning opportunities for a child when working with an adult, and thereby lead to different outcomes.

To explore whether the goal of social interaction influences the way in which adults interact with children during joint planning, Gauvain (1995) used the grocery store task to study the behavior of mothers and 3½- to 5½-year-old children as they planned together. Two experimental conditions were compared: half of the dyads were told prior to the interaction that there was a subsequent individual posttest for the child (aware condition) and half of the dyads were not forewarned of the posttest (unaware condition).

During the interaction participants in both the aware and the unaware conditions were equally successful at planning. However, the way in which the partners in these two conditions coordinated responsibility during the task differed. Dyads who were aware of the posttest shared more responsibility during joint planning than their counterparts who were not aware. Furthermore, for the parts of the task when the partners did not share responsibility, mothers who were not aware of the posttest did more of the planning on their own without the children's help. These patterns suggest that when dyads are aware of a child-only posttest, children are more involved in the task, presumably because they feel that this will help them prepare for the upcoming independent trial.

These findings are consistent with those from other research that shows that participants organize their behavior in relation to the goal of the activity (Renshaw & Gardner, 1990; Rogoff, Ellis, & Gardner, 1984). When there is an instructional goal, the way in which the partners interact differs from when they do not have such a goal. This suggests that guided participation (Rogoff, 1990) may be enhanced when particular activity goals are operative. Are there other social aspects of joint planning that may influence what children learn from planning with adults? To answer this question we turn to an examination of the role of shared social history in parent–child interaction.

Shared Social History and Joint Planning

When children and parents, or in fact any partners, work together on a cognitive task, it is important to consider whether the partners have had prior experience with one another. Shared social history may regulate the cognitive opportunities that arise during joint activity and this, in turn, may affect what children learn from these experiences.

To explore this issue, Gauvain and DeMent (1991) examined how one aspect of child behavior, the child's history of compliance with parental requests, was related to the process of joint cognitive activity on a route-planning task. A history of child noncompliance was identified as an ideal forum for examining the linkages between prior interactional experience, cognitive guidance, and opportunities during a joint cognitive activity to develop cognitive skill. Although the balance of parental requests and child responsivity shifts by situational demands, the requirements of instructional encounters, in particular, may elicit compliance difficulties for parents and children. In an ideal learning situation, such as that described as occurring in the zone of proximal development (Vygotsky, 1978), regulation of task materials and process is gradually transferred from the expert to the novice as the novice's skill and understanding increase. But for parents of children considered noncompliant this process may proceed quite differently.

Mother–child dyads involving 4- to 5-year-old children, half of whom were identified as noncompliant and half of whom had compliance behaviors in the normal range, were observed as they interacted on a series of route-planning tasks. Results indicated that the cognitive interaction proceeded quite differently for mothers working with children identified as noncompliant than for those who had compliant children. Mothers of children identified as noncompliant provided a lower level of cognitive assistance and were more directive and negative toward their children than mothers of children identified as compliant. Concern with controlling the child's behavior apparently superseded instructional goals. This research underscores the importance of examining shared social history as a factor in order to understand the connection between social interaction, cognitive opportunity, and cognitive growth.

Although this point was identified in research with children in the years of early childhood and in relation to a particular social behavior, child compliance, it raises interesting questions as to how shared social history may relate to children's opportunity to learn in social context, especially in a context involving familiar social partners. In a 1985 paper, Scribner outlined Vygotsky's concern with the influence of history on psychological development. One of Vygotsky's concerns was how the child's individual history, like the child's current ability, relates to social–cognitive experience. This is, in large part, what is described as the child's contribution when adults and children participate in the child's zone of proximal development. The study by Gauvain and DeMent (1992) extends this point by suggesting that the contribution of the dyad's history is also important. In order to understand a child's behavior and opportunities in social interaction on a cognitive task, it is important to know something about his or her history of social interaction. These data also illustrate that shared social history is not benign (Goodnow, 1987). In some cases, it may open doors as teachers and learners grow together. In others, it may be more like building among the ruins, as partners rely on wobbly pilings and old materials. Shared social history is an inextricable aspect of human development. Coming to know, in large part, entails coming to know the other and learning with them.

Planning with an Adult versus Planning with a "Trained" Peer Revisited

Is there something unique about adult guidance or could a peer, with appropriate training, provide similar learning experiences for children? In other words, is it the cognitive contact per se that explains better posttest performance, or is there some other feature of adult–child interaction that also contributes? Radziszewska and Rogoff (1991) examined this question by observing the planning of 9- to 11-year-old children as they planned with a peer partner who was trained, prior to the interaction, to use the optimal strategy for doing the task. This research also included adult–child and untrained peer conditions for comparison purposes. The optimal strategy was derived from results of an earlier study of adult–child interaction on this same task (Radziszewska & Rogoff, 1991).

These researchers found that training a peer did not help produce the same type of social experience that children have when they interact with an adult. Children who worked with either a trained or an untrained peer produced less effective plans on the posttest than children who planned with an adult. This appeared to have been due to the children's participation in decision making during the interactional session. Children who planned with adults were more actively involved in decision making during the task than those who planned with a peer, trained or untrained. Furthermore, only adult partners explained the optimal strategy when they used it. When peer partners used this strategy, they did not talk about it.

Thus, planning with adults involved more explicit attention to planning strategies and more active involvement by the children in the planning process. These results indicate that adults are not only more skilled than trained peers at planning, they are also better at communicating this skill to children during joint activity. In addition, adults are better at collaborating with a partner because they encourage more active involvement from children. This finding is related to the research discussed previously regarding the important role that sharing responsibility for decision making plays in regulating children's opportunities to learn from social interaction. It also indicates that two important skills, task explanation and communicative competence, are intricately involved in children's opportunities to learn about planning from social experience. Both of these are more likely to occur when adults and children plan together than when peers—even peers trained in the optimal strategy—engage in joint planning.

CONCLUDING THOUGHTS

The ability to plan, to guide future actions in ways that meet desired goals, is a hallmark of the human intellect in various domains. This chapter began with a description of a remarkable type of planning, Incan quipus. Little is known about how children or apprentices in the ancient Incan Empire learned to plan out messages using this complex communication system. What research on children's planning suggests is that this was very likely a long-term, socially based, learning process involving novices and experts. In the modern world, children have many opportunities to learn about planning from others, both adults and other children. Children are active agents in this process as their developing social, emotional, linguistic, and cognitive skills support and constrain their efforts to learn. Because of its complexity, both in terms of its reliance on many cognitive skills and its need to be adapted to the circumstances at hand, planning takes a fairly long time for children to learn. In addition to learning how to plan actions to reach their goals, children need to develop skills for conveying and coordinating their plans with others. This learning occurs in social context as more experienced planners help steer the course of development of children's planning skills.

Children, especially during early and middle childhood, benefit from planning with others. What children learn from planning differs depending on whether their partner is an adult or another child. In large part this is due to the social–cognitive processes that emerge when children plan with these two types of partners. Adults provide children with more overt and explicit opportunities to learn about task structure, which is common in adult–child interaction when children are in the preschool years. Adults provide more information about planning strategies for children in the years of middle childhood. Adults are more successful than peers in helping children learn about planning because they are more likely to verbalize the thinking process they use during planning and because of their better skills at social coordination.

Peer influence on the development of planning rarely appears as overt instruction. Rather, it is a more implicit process that emerges from children's efforts to coordinate plans with each another. Because the planning process is less overt when peers plan together than when children plan with adults, it appears that the consequences of planning (or not) are especially important in helping children learn about planning from experience with age mates. Experience planning with peers seems to be particularly valuable in providing children with opportunities to learn and practice social planning strategies, like how to decide on and negotiate activities—skills that are essential to both social and cognitive development.

Certain features of the social context contribute in important ways to children's opportunities to learn about planning from social interaction. Some of these provide an indirect form of support that mediates children's limited capacities in other domains relevant to planning. Script knowledge is an interesting example in this regard. Social conventions for organizing information, like scripts, appear to mediate the memory load of planning, which is especially helpful for younger children. Other social aspects, such as the activity goal and the prior experience the partners have had with one another, also play a role in defining what children learn about planning in social context.

Chapter 8

Conclusions and Future Directions

*I*n *The Divine Comedy* Dante asks the question "What do we need in order to grow?" (Mayes, 1996). This is a question about development. In many ways the answer given by developmentalists differs from that of Dante. After all, he was on a moral journey, one he felt was necessary in order for him to become a better person. But, interestingly, the mechanism Dante saw as underlying his passage is not unlike the one proposed by developmental psychologists who adopt a social approach to cognitive development. For Dante, other people—those he encountered on his journey—provided guidance and direction along the way. In a sociocultural approach to cognitive development, the human community guides the intellectual journey that children take over the years of childhood.

Throughout the history of the field, psychologists have primarily studied cognition and its development in laboratory settings where individuals engage in cognitive activity on their own. Yet cognitive development as it actually occurs is nested in a social world that contains historical, contemporary, and prospective influences. All of these define and steer the course of cognitive growth. This process is most evident as older and more experienced members of a community interact with younger, less experienced community members in the course of intelligent action. This process serves many purposes. It ensures that children learn the practices, values, and goals of the community as they move toward maturity. Thus, it serves the child by guiding his or her developing capabilities in meaningful and valued ways. It serves the community in that it connects generations over time, and children and families in communities to one another. The social context of cognitive development links intellectual activity and its development directly to its social and historical foundations.

No single study discussed in this book is sufficient to support the thesis that the social context of development, instantiated in the interaction of its members, is a mechanism of cognitive growth. However, collectively, the research discussed here tells a very compelling story. This research suggests that in order to understand intellectual development, it is essential to examine the role that social experience plays in this process, as well as how, over the course of development, the social world becomes a constituent element of individual functioning. Children have much to learn over the course of growth. The influences they have in this development are many and varied. Research indicates that social interaction with more experienced partners, as Vygotsky (1978) suggested, influences both the content and the process of cognitive development—that is, it affects what children learn to think about and how they come to think about these things. The emotional context of development plays an important role in this process as it guides human motivation, interest, and affect. In addition, the emotional connection between children and those who guide their learning affects the nature and extent of learning and development that occurs in social context. The main processes by which the social world supports, leads, and constrains cognitive growth that were examined in this research are scaffolding, guided participation, instruction, and legitimate peripheral participation. All of these communicate new ways of knowing to the child. They are effective because they are targeted toward the child's region of sensitivity for growth.

This brings us to the question with which we began: Is the social context, as instantiated in these social interactional processes, a mechanism of cognitive change? The research discussed in this book suggests that most of the basic criteria that need to be met in order to qualify as a mechanism of change (Miller, 1993) are satisfied by these social processes. I now consider each criterion in turn.

The social interactional processes listed above, but especially scaffolding and guided participation, incorporate as a central, defining feature the antecedents required for change. This is because these processes are defined by and coordinated with the current (or presenting) capabilities of the child and his or her developmental trajectory in a particular domain. In other words, these social interactional processes are predicated on the fit between what the child already knows and where the interaction is designed to lead him or her. And, as research shows, these processes are only effective when this condition is met.

A second criterion needed in order for a process to qualify as a mechanism of developmental change is the inclusion of a motivating force or forces that generate the change. In a sociocultural approach, both the social agents and the target child involved in the process are motivated similarly. Social agents are motivated to enact change in the hope of making the child increasingly adapted to the circumstances of growth. The child is similarly motivated so that he or she fits in with the environment, especially the social world. More experienced and trusted people, like parents, are gold mines for children in this regard. It is important to point out that this type of motivation is the same as that which appears in Piaget's and many other developmental theories, as Siegler (1996) has discussed.

A third criterion necessary for a process to qualify as a mechanism of change is some specification of factors that may modify change in individual cases. Much of the research discussed in the preceding chapters has as its focus the characteristics of the child, the partner, or the dyad that may influence the nature and course of social–cognitive activity. Research suggests that many of these characteristics may operate in a principled way to regulate the process and outcome of cognitive interaction. However, more study is needed to specify these factors in terms of how they modify intellectual development.

A mechanism of change must also explain why certain courses of development occur and others do not. From the vantage point of a social–contextual view, the answer to this, at present, is painted in very broad strokes. It includes ideas about why certain cognitive changes emerge in some contexts and not in others. Goodnow's (1990) call for research on the ways in which cultural values organize and regulate opportunities for cognitive development in social context is prescient in this regard. Further research would shed much light on this topic.

Another criterion pertains to the ways in which a mechanism facilitates the development of new skills. Numerous illustrations of this process were discussed in the four domains of development that were examined more closely. In early attention, social experience facilitates how children learn to allocate their attentional skills across several sources of information in the environment (e.g., object and mother), as well as how infants evaluate incoming information (social referencing). In early memory development, social experience influences how children encode information in memory, as well as the content knowledge they develop and the strategies they have available for storing, retrieving, and sharing these memories. In both problem solving and planning, the main input from the social world is in the areas of strategy acquisition and selection. Together, this evidence suggests that processes that emerge from social experience facilitate in unique ways the development of new skills in several domains of intellectual growth.

Finally, a complete account of a mechanism of developmental change should include evidence of how cognitive skills are accessed in specific contexts as well as evidence of how cognitive skills are transferred from one context to another. Little research on the social context of cognitive development has investigated these topics. The few studies that do examine the transfer of skills that were learned in one context to very similar problem situations (e.g., the pretest–interaction–posttest design). In these studies, as in research on individual development that uses a similar design but with the intervening step being some type of task experience that is not social (like practice), improvements in performance are observed. Transfer to a different context of performance or over a longer period of time has not been the object of sufficient study. It is important to stress that research using a social–contextual approach is no more remiss in this regard than cognitive developmental research based on more individual approaches, like neo-Piagetian or information-processing views. Examination of transfer requires further study in all the approaches currently used in the field.

In sum, the social context of cognitive development satisfies many of the criteria considered important in order for a process to be considered a mechanism of change. Although further study is needed, results to date support this assertion.

In order to examine the social context as a mechanism of cognitive change, I discussed the three primary social agents involved in this process. These are the family, peers, and life in the community, though my emphasis was primarily on family and peer influences. This is because the contribution that life in the community makes to cognitive development has not been the focus of much systematic research. Much more attention to this influence is needed.

In regards to the family, special attention was paid to the role that parents play in children's cognitive development. Parent–child relations have long been recognized as an early and highly influential context for socialization. Most of the research on this topic has focused on parental socialization in the areas of child social behavior. However, as the research discussed here shows, a literature on parental influences on cognitive development in many areas of cognition is emerging. Although much of this research has concentrated on mother–child interaction, fathers and even siblings are increasingly the focus of study. In addition, both direct and indirect parental influences are important to cognitive development, though more research evidence exists on direct than indirect influences. *Direct influences* are those that occur during social interaction. *Indirect influences* include parents' role in managing and arranging specific opportunities for children to develop cognitive skills, such as out-of-school lessons, computer use at home, monitoring of children's homework and other learning opportunities, and initiating and arranging children's activities that involve intelligent behavior—for example, through clubs and types of informal play that require planning and problem solving. In terms of development, the direct and indirect influences on cognitive development that parents provide are related to child age. As research has shown, much of the influence that parents have over cognitive development in the early years of childhood is through processes of direct interaction. During middle childhood, as children's social life expands, indirect parental influences are increasingly influential. During middle childhood, one of the primary social influences on children's cognitive development is peers. Research shows that peers provide important opportunities for cognitive development in the classroom, through cooperative learning and peer tutoring, and outside the classroom, through play, joint problem solving, and collaborative activity. Research also suggests that peer influence on cognitive development is mediated by a number of factors, including expertise, social roles, age, and gender. Further examination of the role that each of these factors plays in various domains of cognitive development would enrich our understanding of the contribution that peers make to intellectual growth during middle childhood.

Four domains of cognitive development—attention, memory, problem solving, and planning—were examined closely in relation to how social experience may contribute to their development in childhood. These domains were each discussed briefly in terms of what is known from research that does not attend to social context, and then each was examined in relation to research that considers social context, especially adult and peer contributions. The research reviewed in these areas of cognitive development paints an intriguing portrait of how social experience contributes to cognitive development. Processes like intersubjectivity, joint attention, social referencing, shared remembering, and joint problem solving and planning compose a substantial part of children's learning experiences. These processes are, by definition, simultaneously social and cognitive. Certainly, the child *brings* capabilities of his or her own to these interactions—this is not contested. But what is important in developmental terms is what a child *takes away* from these experiences.

The research discussed suggests that the course of intellectual growth in each of these domains is affected by social experience in meaningful ways. Evidence includes the fact that infants learn much about how to deploy their attentional skills from others, that toddlers and preschoolers seek and process the evaluations that others have concerning information in the environment, that preschoolers and early school-age children rehearse and retain knowledge and memories that are considered valuable and important to others, and that children, especially in the years of middle childhood, learn about ways of remembering and solving problems and planning the future from others. Together, these observations suggest that a lion's share of the higher level cognitive functions that children develop in the early to middle years of childhood are intricately connected to social experience.

In addition to theoretical issues, there are also practical reasons for examining the social context of cognitive development. Such research may help address questions about variation in cognitive development within and across social and cultural communities. Furthermore, by examining social context and cognitive development as constituent factors, it may be possible to discern what aspects of cognitive development are universal or biologically determined and what aspects are influenced by social and cultural context. Traditional approaches to cognitive development that propose universal modes of functioning are limited in addressing this issue because they tend to frame children's performance relative to either an absolute standard or to a standard that is descriptive of one pattern of development, typically that of middle-class European American children. This has led to deficit models of intelligence that suggest that those who do not meet the standard are deficient in some way. This approach is not only based on faulty reasoning, it can also be used in support of social injustice. An approach to cognitive development that incorporates social context as part of cognitive growth can help psychologists better address this issue.

In terms of future directions for research, there are many areas that need attention if we are to obtain a more complete understanding of the social context of cognitive development. This effort will be expedited if findings from studies that adopt a social–contextual approach are reconciled and coordinated with research findings in these same domains of study that did not take a social approach. For example, how does the extensive research on children's theory of mind that is based on children's individual performance on various types of tasks relate to the social and cultural context in which these skills develop, including the emergence and support for a type of reasoning and communication that is a critical aspect of this area of study?

This question implies that even research that has attempted to minimize or ignore the role of social and cultural experience on children's cognitive performance still has social and cultural processes embedded in the performances that are observed. In fact, even research conducted under the most controlled and seemingly nonsocial of conditions reflects social and cultural influences. For example, if a research participant can understand what he or she is being asked to do in a study and he or she participates in the study in a meaningful way, then the research is conducted in a social context. This is because the individual's performance relies on the shared meaning that the investigator and the participant bring to the research context. Recognition of this fact does not undermine the individual internal contributions that participants bring to the study. It simply points out that the individual performance is supported by social and cultural experiences that created the "sense making" that occurred and made this research possible. More understanding is needed of how this sense-making ability comes about and the role it plays in cognitive performance and development. However, as this example suggests, it is often difficult to detect where individual contributions stop and social and cultural contributions begin. In sum, examination of research in terms of what participants are trying to do may help clarify how the social context contributes to cognitive development in specific domains, as well as elucidate what children need to know in order to participate in the research. Of course, methods to do this need to be devised, and these need to satisfy psychologists' standards of scientific rigor and demonstration. An activity-based approach, such as that suggested by Leont'ev (1981), but adapted to the study of development, may be useful in this regard.

I hope that the chapters in which I examine specific areas of cognitive development illustrate that any psychological performance may be affected by the social and cultural context of growth. It is also the case though that, to the benefit of the organism but to the bane of researchers, social and cultural contributions are often invisible and easy to overlook. The seamless connection between individual social and mental life supports everyday functioning in many ways. Therefore, the task for researchers is to make the invisible visible, and to do so without causing too great an impact on the behavior under scrutiny (i.e., experimenter effects). A next step in this direction may be the specification of how the social context can influence specific areas of intellectual growth at particular points in development. Contextual approaches, such as Bronfenbrenner's (1979), provide guidance in this direction, as does sociocultural theory (discussed in Part I of this book).

In conclusion, several points are stressed in this book. First and foremost is the idea that the adoption of a sociocultural view of cognitive development enhances understanding of the process of intellectual growth. It does so by providing information about cognitive development that is unique relative to the main approaches in the field. Thus, a sociocultural view complements contemporary research, including neo-Piagetian and information-processing views. A second important point is that dimensions of the social context of cognitive development are realized in intelligent human activity. It is possible to specify and study these in relation to psychological development. These dimensions can help bring the social and cultural character of human intellectual development into relief, and thereby help researchers "see the social and the cultural" in individual psychological development. Third, better understanding of the social context of cognitive development can be advanced by the reexamination of findings on individual development in the literature. If, as theory suggests, social and cultural life play a role in all human psychological functioning, it would be foolhardy to dismiss a long history of careful research because social influences on the process was not taken explicitly into account.

All this said, many hard questions remain. One of these concerns how to understand and describe individual skill that emerges in and is displayed in social situations. Although some may argue that individual analysis is anathema to a sociocultural approach—and this may be true in a philosophical or theoretical sense—a conceptualization that allows the investigator who holds a sociocultural view to locate individual thinking and individual contributions within social processes is sorely needed. Psychologists have yet to devise a language for describing thinking that is not entirely in the head of the child or, in other words, only partially in place. Haith (1997) discusses this point in a recent paper examining infant cognition. His arguments are relevant here. He points out that the study and description of intellectual accomplishments are typically based on an all-or-nothing view of cognitive processes. That is, many of the cognitive skills that children develop are defined in dichotomous terms. Consider mental representations. Representations are typically understood as something that a person either has or does not have. In other words, mental representations are conceptualized as *states* of understanding rather than as *processes* of understanding, and rarely as something that is partially or incompletely achieved. Such conceptualization may suffice in describing the mature thinker in any particular domain, though even this is an open question. But it is surely inadequate for describing the development of knowledge that appears in the form of "partial understanding," such as that located in social performance. Thus, in order to incorporate the notion of partial or socially contextualized intellectual accomplishments into an understanding of cognitive development and learning, a different conceptualization of many cognitive skills is needed. The view offered by Rogoff (1998) of development as a process of changing roles and responsibilities in the course of social participation is promising in this regard.

A second hard question pertains to the role that cognitive developmental psychologists can play in certain national discussions. One need not be a fortune teller to know that analyses of culture and ethnicity in all aspects of psychological functioning will increase dramatically in the next decade. The current social, political, and intellectual climate is consumed by these issues. What role will developmental psychology or psychology more generally play in this process? It is hard to say. I would like to see developmental psychology play a significant role because I believe it can bring interesting, important, and unique insights to the discussion. However, I also feel that in many ways the field is currently ill-equipped to do this. Perhaps by developing conceptual frameworks, frameworks in which social and cultural systems of interacting and supporting thinking are an inextricable part of cognitive development, developmental psychologists will be able to contribute to this important debate.

References

Adamson, L. B. (1995). *Communication development during infancy.* Madison, WI: Brown & Benchmark.

Adamson, L. B., & Bakeman, R. (1985). Affect and attention: Infants observed with mothers and peers. *Child Development, 56,* 582–593.

Adamson, L. B., & Bakeman, R. (1991). The development of shared attention during infancy. In R. Vasta (Ed.), *Annals of child development* (Vol. 8, pp. 1–41). London: Kingsley.

Adamson, L. B., & McArthur, D. (1995). Joint attention, affect, and culture. In C. Moore & P. J. Dunham (Eds.), *Joint attention: Its origins and role in development* (pp. 205–221). Hillsdale, NJ: Erlbaum.

Aktar, N., Dunham, F., & Dunham, P. (1991). Directive interactions and early vocabulary development: The role of joint attentional focus. *Journal of Child Language, 18,* 41–49.

Altman, I., & Rogoff, B. (1987). World views in psychology: Trait, interactional, organismic, and transactional perspectives. In D. Stokols & I. Altman (Eds.), *Handbook of environmental psychology* (Vol. 1, pp. 7–40). New York: Wiley.

Altmann, J. (1974). Observational study of behavior: Sampling methods. *Behavior, 49,* 227–265.

Anderson, D. R., Choi, H. P., & Lorch, E. P. (1987). Attentional inertia reduces distractibility during young children's TV viewing. *Child Development, 58,* 798–806.

Angelou, M. (1969). *I know why the caged bird sings.* New York: Bantam Books.

Ascher, M., & Ascher, R. (1981). *The code of the Quipu: A study in media, mathematics, and culture.* Ann Arbor: University of Michigan Press.

Ascher, M., & Ascher, R. (1997). *Mathematics of the Incas: Code of the Quipu.* Minneola, NY: Dover.

Ashmead, D. H., & Perlmutter, M. (1980). Infant memory in everyday life. In M. Perlmutter (Ed.), *Children's memory* (pp. 1–16). San Francisco: Jossey-Bass.

Astington, J. W. (1993). *The child's discovery of the mind.* Cambridge, MA: Harvard University Press.

Azmitia, M. (1987, April). *Expertise as a moderator of social influence on children's cognition.* Paper presented at the meeting of the Society for Research in Child Development, Baltimore.

Azmitia, M. (1988). Peer interaction and problem solving: When are two heads better than one? *Child Development, 59,* 87–96.

Azmitia, M., & Hesser, J. (1993). Why siblings are important agents of cognitive development: A comparison of siblings and peers. *Child Development, 64,* 430–444.

Azmitia, M., & Montgomery, R. (1993). Friendship, transactive dialogues, and the development of scientific reasoning. *Social Development, 2,* 202–221.

Azmitia, M., & Perlmutter, M. (1989). Social influences on children's cognition: State of the art and future directions. In H. Reese (Ed.), *Advances in child development and behavior* (Vol. 22, pp. 89–144). Orlando, FL: Academic Press.

Bakeman, R., & Adamson, L. B. (1984). Coordinating attention to people and objects in mother-infant and peer–infant interaction. *Child Development, 55,* 1278–1289.

Bakeman, R., Adamson, L. B., Konner, M., & Barr, R. G. (1990). !Kung infancy: The social context of object exploration. *Child Development, 61,* 794–809.

Baldwin, D. A. (1991). Infants' contribution to the achievement of joint reference. *Child Development, 62,* 875–890.

Bandura, A. (1977). *Social learning theory.* Englewood Cliffs, NJ: Prentice-Hall.

Bandura, A. (1986). *Social foundations of thought and action: A social cognitive theory.* Englewood Cliffs, NJ: Prentice-Hall.

Barrett, K. C. (1985). Infants' use of conflicting emotion signals (Doctoral dissertation, University of Denver, 1984). *Dissertation Abstracts International, 46,* 321B–322B.

Bartlett, F. C. (1932). *Remembering: A study in experimental and social psychology.* Cambridge, UK: Cambridge University Press.

Bartlett, F. C. (1958). *Thinking: An experimental and social study.* New York: Basic Books.

Bauer, P. J., & Mandler, J. M. (1990). Remembering what happened next: Very young children's recall of event sequences. In R. Fivush & J. A. Hudson (Eds.), *Knowing and remembering in young children* (pp. 9–29). Cambridge, UK: Cambridge University Press.

Benson, J. B. (1994). The origins of future orientation in the everyday lives of 9- to 36-month-old infants. In M. M. Haith, J. B. Benson, R. J. Roberts, & B. F. Pennington (Eds.), *The development of future-oriented processes* (pp. 375–407). Chicago: University of Chicago Press.

Benson, J. B., & Haith, M. (1995). Future-oriented processes: A foundation for planning behavior in infants and toddlers. *Infancia y Aprendizaje, 69–70,* 127–140.

Bertenthal, B. I. (1993). Perception of biomechanical motions by infants: Intrinsic image and knowledge-based constraints. In C. E. Granrud (Ed.), *Visual perception and cognition in infancy* (pp. 175–214). Hillsdale, NJ: Erlbaum.

Bertenthal, B. I., & Campos, J. J. (1990). A systems approach to the organizing efforts of self-produced locomotion during infancy. In C. K. Rovee-Collier & L. Lipsitt (Eds.), *Advances in infancy research* (Vol. 6, pp. 1–60). Norwood, NJ: Ablex.

Best, D. L., & Ornstein, P. A. (1986). Children's generation and communication of mnemonic strategies. *Developmental Psychology, 22,* 845–853.

Bjorkland, D. F. (1990). *Children's strategies: Contemporary views of cognitive development.* Hillsdale, NJ: Erlbaum

Blurton Jones, N. (1972). *Ethological studies of child behavior.* London: Cambridge University Press.

Bransford, J. D., & Franks, J. J. (1972). The abstraction of linguistic ideas: A review. *Cognition, 1,* 211–249.

Brazelton, T. B., Koslowski, B., & Main, M. (1974). The origins of reciprocity: The early mother–infant interaction. In M. Lewis & L. A. Rosenblum (Eds.), *The origins of behavior: The effect of the infant on its caregiver* (pp. 49–76). New York: Wiley.

Bretherton, I. (1992). Social referencing, intentional communication, and the interfacing of minds in infancy. In S. Feinman (Ed.), *Social referencing and the social construction of reality in infancy* (pp. 57–77). New York: Plenum Press.

Bronfenbrenner, U. (1979). *The ecology of human development.* Cambridge, MA: Harvard University Press.

Bronfenbrenner, U. (1986). Recent advances in research on the ecology of human development. In R. K. Silvereisen, K. Eyferth, & G. Rudinger (Eds.), *Development as action in context* (pp. 286–309). New York: Springer-Verlag.

Brown, A. L., Bransford, J. D., Ferrara, R. A., & Campione, J. C. (1983). Learning, remembering, and understanding. In J. H. Flavell & E. M. Markman (Eds.), *Handbook of child psychology* (Vol. 3, pp. 515–629). New York: Wiley.

Brown, A. L., & Campione, J. C. (1984). Three faces of transfer: Implications for early competence, individual differences, and instruction. In M. E. Lamb & A. L. Brown (Eds.), *Advances in developmental psychology* (Vol. 3, pp. 143–192). Hillsdale, NJ: Erlbaum.

Brown, A. L., & DeLoache, J. S. (1978). Skills, plans, and self-regulation. In R. S. Siegler (Ed.), *Children's thinking: What develops?* (pp. 3–35). Hillsdale, NJ: Erlbaum.

Brownell, C. A., & Carriger, M. S. (1991). Collaborations among toddler peers: Individual contributions to social contexts. In L. B. Resnick, J. M. Levine, & S. D. Teasley (Eds.), *Perspectives on socially shared cognition* (pp. 365–383). Washington, DC: American Psychological Association.

Bruner, J. S. (1975). The ontogenesis of speech acts. *Journal of Child Language, 1,* 1–19.

Bruner, J. S. (1982). The organization of action and the nature of adult–infant interaction. In E. Z. Tronick (Ed.), *Social interchange in infancy: Affect, cognition, and communication* (pp. 23–35). Baltimore: University Park Press.

Bruner, J. S. (1985). Vygotsky: A historical and conceptual perspective. In J. V. Wertsch (Ed.), *Culture, communication, and cognition: Vygotskian perspectives* (pp. 21–34). Cambridge, UK: Cambridge University Press.

Bruner, J. S. (1986). *Actual minds, possible worlds.* Cambridge, MA: Harvard University Press.

Bruner, J. S. (1990). *Acts of meaning.* Cambridge, MA: Harvard University Press.

Bruner, J. S. (1995). From joint attention to the meeting of minds: An introduction. In C. Moore & P. J. Dunham (Eds.), *Joint attention: Its origins and role in development* (pp. 1–14). Hillsdale, NJ: Erlbaum.

Bruner, J. S., & Sherwood, V. (1976). Early rule structure: The case of "peekaboo." In R. Harre (Ed.), *Life sentences* (pp. 55–62). London: Wiley.

Bugental, D. B., & Goodnow, J. J. (1998). Socialization processes. In W. Damon (Series Ed.) & N. Eisenberg (Vol. Ed.), *Handbook of child psychology: Vol. 3. Social, emotional, and personality development* (pp. 389–462). New York: Wiley.

Butterworth, G. (1995). Origins of mind in perception and action. In C. Moore & P. J. Dunham (Eds.), *Joint attention: Its origins and role in development* (pp. 29–40). Hillsdale, NJ: Erlbaum.

Callanan, M. A., & Oakes, L. M. (1992). Preschoolers' questions and parents' explanations: Causal thinking in everyday activity. *Cognitive Development, 7,* 213–233.

Campos, J. J., & Stenberg, C. R. (1981). Perception, appraisal, and emotion: The onset of social referencing. In M. E. Lamb & L. R. Sherrod (Eds.), *Infant social cognition: Empirical and theoretical considerations* (pp. 273–314). Hillsdale, NJ: Erlbaum.

Carpenter, M., Nagell, K., & Tomasello, M. (1998). Social cognition, joint attention, and communicative competence from 9 to 15 months of age. *Monographs of the Society for Research in Child Development, 63* (Serial No. 255). Chicago: University of Chicago Press.

Carraher, T. N., Carraher, D. W., & Schliemann, A. D. (1985). Mathematics in the streets and in schools. *British Journal of Developmental Psychology, 3,* 21–29.

Case, R. (1992). *The mind's staircase: Exploring the conceptual underpinnings of children's thought and knowledge.* Hillsdale, NJ: Erlbaum.

Chatwin, B. (1987). *Songlines.* New York: Viking.

Chavajay, P., & Rogoff, B. (1999). Cultural variation in management of attention by children and their caregivers. *Child Development, 35,* 1079–1090.

Chi, M. T. H. (1978). Knowledge structures and memory development. In R. S. Siegler (Ed.), *Children's thinking: What develops?* (pp. 73–96). Hillsdale, NJ: Erlbaum.

Cohn, J. F., & Tronick, E. Z. (1983). Three-month-old infants' reaction to simulated maternal depression. *Child Development, 54,* 185–193.

Cole, M. (1985). The zone of proximal development: Where culture and cognition create each other. In J. V. Wertsch (Ed.), *Culture, communication, and cognition: Vygotskian perspectives* (pp. 146–161). New York: Cambridge University Press.

Cole, M. (1996). *Cultural psychology: A once and future discipline.* Cambridge, MA: Harvard University Press.

Cole, M., & Cole, S. (1996). *The development of children* (3rd ed.). New York: Freeman.

Cole, M., Gay, J., Glick, J. A., & Sharp, D. W. (1971). *The cultural context of learning and thinking.* New York: Basic Books.

Cole, M., Sharp, D. W., & Lave, C. (1976). The cognitive consequences of education. *Urban Review, 9,* 218–233.

Collie, R., & Hayne, H. (1999). Deferred imitation by 6- and 9-month-old infants: More evidence for declarative memory. *Developmental Psychobiology, 35*, 83–90.

Conner, D. B., Knight, D. K., & Cross, D. R. (1997). Mothers' and fathers' scaffolding of their 2-year-olds during problem solving and literacy interactions. *British Journal of Developmental Psychology, 15*, 323–338.

Cooper, C. R. (1980). Development of collaborative problem solving among preschool children. *Developmental Psychology, 16*, 433–440.

Costanzo, P. R. (1991). Morals, mothers, and memories: The social context of developing social cognition. In R. Cohen & A. W. Siegel (Eds.), *Context and development* (pp. 91–132). Hillsdale, NJ: Erlbaum.

Curtiss, S. (1977). *Genie: A psychological study of a modern-day wild child.* New York: Academic Press.

Damon, W. (1984). Peer education: The untapped potential. *Journal of Applied Developmental Psychology, 5*, 331–343.

Dannemiller, J. L., & Stephens, B. R. (1988). A critical test of infant pattern perception. *Child Development, 59*, 210–216.

Das, J. P., Kar, B. C., & Parrila, R. K. (1996). *Cognitive planning: The psychological basis of intelligent behavior.* New Delhi, India: Sage.

Davidson, D. (1996). The effects of decision characteristics on children's selective search of predecisional information. *Acta Psychologica, 92*, 263–281.

de Beauvoir, S. (1959). *Memoirs of a dutiful daughter.* New York: Harper & Row.

DeCasper, A. J., & Spence, M. J. (1986). Prenatal maternal speech influences newborns' perception of speech sounds. *Infant Behavior and Development, 9*, 133–150.

DeLoache, J. S., Cassidy, D. J., & Brown, A. L. (1985). Precursors of mnemonic strategies in very young children's memory. *Child Development, 56*, 125–137.

Doise, W., Mugny, G., & Perret-Clermont, A. (1975). Social interaction and the development of cognitive operations. *European Journal of Social Psychology, 5*, 367–383.

Donald, M. (1991). *Origins of the modern mind: Three stages in the evolution of culture and cognition.* Cambridge, MA: Harvard University Press.

Donaldson, M. (1978). *Children's minds.* New York: Norton.

Duncker, K. (1945). On problem solving. *Psychological Monographs, 58*(270).

Dunham, P. J., Dunham, F., & Curwin, A. (1993). Joint-attentional states and lexical acquisition at 18 months. *Developmental Psychology, 29*, 827–831.

Dunham, P. J., & Moore, C. (1995). Current themes in research on joint attention. In C. Moore & P. J. Dunham (Eds.), *Joint attention: Its origins and role in development* (pp. 15–28). Hillsdale, NJ: Erlbaum.

Duran, R. T., & Gauvain, M. (1993). The role of age versus expertise in peer collaboration during joint planning. *Journal of Experimental Child Psychology, 55*, 227–242.

Eimas, P. D., Siqueland, E. R., Juscyk, P., & Vigorito, J. (1971). Speech perception in infants. *Science, 171*, 303–306.

Eisenberg, A. R. (1985). Learning to describe past experiences in conversation. *Discourse Processes, 8*, 177–204.

Elder, G. H. (1999). *Children of the Great Depression: Social change in life experience.* Boulder, CO: Westview Press.

Ellis, S. (1995, April). *Social influences on strategy choice.* Paper presented at the meetings of the Society for Research in Child Development, Indianapolis.

Ellis, S., & Gauvain, M. (1992). Social and cultural influences on children's collaborative interactions. In L. T. Winegar & J. Valsiner (Eds.), *Children's development within social context: Research and methodology* (Vol. 2, pp. 155–180). Hillsdale, NJ: Erlbaum.

Ellis, S., Klahr, D., & Siegler, R. S. (1993, March). *Effects of feedback and collaboration on changes in children's use of mathematical rules.* Paper presented at the meeting of the Society for Research in Child Development, New Orleans.

Ellis, S., & Rogoff, B. (1982). The strategies and efficacy of child versus adult teachers. *Child Development, 53,* 730–735.

Engel, S. (1986). *Learning to reminisce: A developmental study of how young children talk about the past.* Unpublished doctoral dissertation, City University of New York Graduate Center, New York.

Engel, S. (1995). *The stories children tell: Making sense of the narratives of childhood.* New York: Freeman.

Fabricius, W. V. (1988). The development of forward search planning in preschoolers. *Child Development, 59,* 1473–1488.

Fagot, B. I., & Gauvain, M. (1997). Mother–child problem solving: Continuity through the childhood years. *Developmental Psychology, 33,* 480–488.

Fagot, B. I., Gauvain, M., & Kavanagh, K. (1996). Infant attachment and mother–child problem solving: A replication. *Journal of Social and Personal Relationships, 13,* 295–302.

Farrar, M. J., & Goodman, G. S. (1992). Developmental changes in event memory. *Child Development, 63,* 173–187.

Feinman, S. (1982). Social referencing in infancy. *Merrill–Palmer Quarterly, 28,* 445–470.

Feinman, S. (1992). *Social referencing and the social construction of reality in infancy.* New York: Plenum Press.

Feinman, S., Roberts, D., Hsieh, K.-F., Sawyer, D., & Swanson, D. (1992). A critical review of social referencing in infancy. In S. Feinman (Ed.), *Social referencing and the social construction of reality in infancy* (pp. 15–54). New York: Plenum Press.

Feldman, N. S., & Ruble, D. N. (1988). The effect of personal relevance on psychological inference: A developmental analysis. *Child Development, 59,* 1339–1352.

Fenson, L., Sapper, V., & Minner, D. G. (1974). Attention and manipulative play in the one-year-old child. *Child Development, 45,* 757–764.

Fernald, A. (1991). Prosody in speech to young children: Prelinguistic and linguistic functions. In R. Vasta (Ed.), *Annals of child development* (Vol. 8, pp. 43–80). London: Kingsley.

Fivush, R. (1988). The functions of event memory: Some comments on Nelson and Brasalou. In U. Neisser & E. Winograd (Eds.), *Remembering reconsidered: Ecological and traditional approaches to the study of memory* (pp. 277–282). New York: Cambridge University Press.

Fivush, R., Haden, C., & Reese, E. (1996). Remembering, recounting, and reminiscing: The development of autobiographical memory in social context. In D. C. Rubin (Ed.), *Remembering our past: Studies in autobiographical memory* (pp. 341–359). Cambridge, UK: Cambridge University Press.

Fivush, R., & Hamond, N. R. (1989). Time and again: Effects of repetition and retention interval on two year olds' event recall. *Journal of Experimental Child Psychology, 47,* 259–273.

Fivush, R., & Hamond, N. R. (1990). Autobiographical memory across the preschool years: Toward reconceptualizing childhood amnesia. In R. Fivush & J. A. Hudson (Eds.), *Knowing and remembering in young children* (pp. 223–248). Cambridge, UK: Cambridge University Press.

Fivush, R., & Hudson, J. A. (Eds.). (1990). *Knowing and remembering in young children.* Cambridge, UK: Cambridge University Press.

Flavell, J. H. (1984). Discussion. In R. J. Sternberg (Ed.), *Mechanisms of cognitive development* (pp. 187–209). New York: Freeman.

Fletcher, K. L., & Bray, N. W. (1996). External memory strategy use in preschool children. *Merrill–Palmer Quarterly, 42,* 379–396.

Foley, M. A., Passalacqua, C., & Ratner, H. H. (1993). Appropriating the actions of another: Implications for children's memory and learning. *Cognitive Development, 8,* 373–401.

Foley, M. A., & Ratner, H. H. (1998). Children's recoding in memory for collaboration: A way of learning from others. *Cognitive Development, 13,* 91–108.

Forbes, D. L., Katz, M. M., Paul, B., & Lubin, D. (1982). Children's plans for joining play: An analysis of structure and function. In D. Forbes & M. T. Greenberg (Eds.), *Children's planning strategies* (pp. 61–79). San Francisco: Jossey-Bass.

Fraiberg, S. H. (1959). *The magic years: Understanding and handling the problems of early childhood.* New York: Scribners.

Frank, A. (1952). *The diary of a young girl.* New York: Modern Library.

Frankel, K. A., & Bates, J. E. (1990). Mother–toddler problem solving: Antecedents in attachment, home behavior, and temperament. *Child Development, 61,* 810–819.

Frankel, M. T., & Rollins, H. A. (1983). Does mother know best? Mothers and fathers interacting with preschool sons and daughters. *Developmental Psychology, 19,* 694–702.

Franklin, B. (1961). *The autobiography and other writings.* New York: Penguin. (Original work published 1771)

Frese, M., & Sabini, J. (1985). *Goal-directed behavior: The concept of action in psychology.* Hillsdale, NJ: Erlbaum.

Freund, L. (1990). Maternal regulation of children's problem solving behavior and its impact on children's performance. *Child Development, 61,* 113–126.

Friedman, S. L., Scholnick, E. K., & Cocking, R. R. (1987). *Blueprints for thinking: The role of planning in psychological development.* Cambridge, UK: Cambridge University Press.

Fuster, J. M. (1989). *The prefrontal cortex* (2nd ed.). New York: Raven Press.

Gathercole, S. E. (1998). The development of memory. *Journal of Child Psychology and Psychiatry and Allied Disciplines, 39,* 3–27.

Gauvain, M. (1989). Children's planning in social context: An observational study of kindergartners' planning in the classroom. In L. T. Winegar (Ed.), *Social interaction and the development of children's understanding* (pp. 95–117). Norwood, NJ: Ablex.

Gauvain, M. (1992). Social influences on the development of planning in advance and during action. *International Journal of Behavioral Development, 15,* 377–398.

Gauvain, M. (1995). Influence of purpose of an interaction on adult–child planning. *Infancia y Aprendizaje, 69–70,* 141–155.

Gauvain, M. (1999). Everyday opportunities for the development of planning skills: Sociocultural and family influences. In A. Goncu (Ed.), *Children's engagement in the world: Sociocultural perspectives* (pp. 173–201). Cambridge, UK: Cambridge University Press.

Gauvain, M., de la Ossa, J., & Hurtado, M. (1996, June). *Social influences on the development of children's skill at reading plans.* Paper presented at the meeting of the Jean Piaget Society, Philadelphia.

Gauvain, M., & DeMent, T. (1991). The role of shared social history in parent–child cognitive activity. *Newsletter of the Laboratory of Comparative Human Cognition, 13,* 58–66.

Gauvain, M., & Fagot, B. I. (1995). Child temperament as a mediator of mother–toddler problem solving. *Social Development, 4,* 257–276.

Gauvain, M., Fagot, B. I., Leve, C., & Kavanagh, K. (2000). *Guidance and support by mothers and fathers within and between families during joint problem solving with young children.* Unpublished manuscript, University of California, Riverside, Department of Psychology.

Gauvain, M., & Huard, R. D. (1999). Family interaction, parenting style, and the development of planning: A longitudinal analysis using archival data. *Journal of Family Psychology, 13,* 1–18.

Gauvain, M., & Rogoff, B. (1989). Collaborative problem solving and children's planning skills. *Developmental Psychology, 25,* 139–151.

Gearhart, M. (1979, March). *Social planning: Role play in a novel situation.* Paper presented at the meeting of the Society for Research in Child Development, San Francisco.

Geertz, C. (1973). *The interpretation of cultures.* New York: Basic Books.

Gelman, R. (1979). Preschool thought. *American Psychologist, 34,* 900–905.

Gelman, R., & Greeno, J. G. (1989). On the nature of competence: Principles for understanding in a domain. In L. B. Resnick (Ed.), *Knowing and learning: Issues for a cognitive science of instruction* (pp. 125–186). Hillsdale, NJ: Erlbaum.

Gelman, R., Massey, C. M., & McManus, M. (1991). Characterizing supporting environments for cognitive development: Lessons from children in a museum. In L. B. Resnick, J. M. Levine, & S. D. Teasley (Eds.), *Perspectives on socially shared cognition* (pp. 226–256). Washington, DC: American Psychological Association.

Gelman, S., Coley, J. D., Rosengren, K. S., Hartman, E., & Pappas, A. (1998). Beyond labeling: The role of maternal input in the acquisition of richly structured categories. *Monographs of the Society for Research in Child Development, 63*(1, Serial No. 253).

Gewirtz, J. L., & Pelaez-Nogueras, M. (1992). Social referencing as a learned process. In S. Feinman (Ed.), *Social referencing and the social construction of reality in infancy* (pp. 151–173). New York: Plenum Press.

Gibson, E., & Rader, N. (1979). Attention: The perceiver as performer. In G. A. Hale & M. Lewis (Eds.), *Attention and cognitive development* (pp. 1–21). New York: Plenum Press.

Gibson, J. J. (1979). *The ecological approach to visual perception.* Boston: Houghton Mifflin.

Gilmore, R. O., & Johnson, M. H. (1995). Working memory in infancy: Six-month-olds' performance on two versions of the oculocomotor delayed response task. *Journal of Experimental Child Psychology, 59,* 397–418.

Glachen, M., & Light, P. (1982). Peer interaction and learning: Can two wrongs make a right? In G. Butterworth & P. Light (Eds.), *Social cognition: Studies of the development of understanding* (pp. 238–262). Brighton, UK: Harvester Press.

Goldman-Rakic, P. S. (1987). Development of cortical circuitry and cognitive function. *Child Development, 58,* 601–622.

Goldsmith, D., & Rogoff, B. (1995). Mothers' and toddlers' coordinated joint focus of attention: Variations with maternal dysphoric symptoms. *Developmental Psychology, 33,* 113–119.

Goncu, A. (1993). Development of intersubjectivity in the dyadic play of preschoolers. *Early Childhood Research Quarterly, 8,* 99–116.

Goodnow, J. J. (1987, November). *The socialization of cognition: Who's involved?* Paper presented at the conference on Culture and Human Development, Chicago.

Goodnow, J. J. (1990). The socialization of cognition: What's involved? In J. W. Stigler, R. A. Shweder, & G. Herdt (Eds.), *Cultural psychology: Essays on comparative human development* (pp. 259–286). Cambridge, UK: Cambridge University Press.

Goodnow, J. J., Miller, P. J., & Kessel, F. (1995). *Cultural practices as contexts for development.* San Francisco: Jossey-Bass.

Goodwin, D. K. (1997). *Wait till next year: A memoir.* New York: Simon & Schuster.

Goody, J. (1977). *The domestication of the savage mind.* Cambridge, UK: Cambridge University Press.

Gottlieb, G. (1992). *Individual development and evolution: The genesis of novel behavior.* New York: Oxford University Press.

Greenfield, P. M. (1980). Toward an operational and logical analysis of intentionality: The use of discourse in early child language. In D. R. Olson (Ed.), *The social foundations of language and thought* (pp. 254–279). New York: Norton.

Greenfield, P. M. (1984). A theory of the teacher in the learning activities of everyday life. In B. Rogoff & J. Lave (Eds.), *Everyday cognition: Its development in social context* (pp. 117–138). Cambridge, MA: Harvard University Press.

Greenfield, P. M., & Childs, C. P. (1991). Developmental continuity in biocultural context. In R. Cohen & A. W. Siegel (Eds.), *Context and development* (pp. 135–159). Hillsdale, NJ: Erlbaum.

Greenfield, P. M., & Lave, J. (1982). Cognitive aspects of informal education. In

D. A. Wagner & H. W. Stevenson (Eds.), *Cultural perspectives on child development* (pp. 208–224). San Francisco: Freeman.

Grusec, J. E., & Lytton, H. (1988). *Social development.* New York: Springer.

Haden, C. A. (1998). Reminiscing with different children: Relating maternal stylistic consistency and sibling similarity in talk about the past. *Child Development, 34,* 99–114.

Haith, M. M. (1994). Visual expectations as the first step toward the development of future-oriented processes. In M. M. Haith, J. B. Benson, R. J. Roberts, & B. F. Pennington (Eds.), *The development of future-oriented processes* (pp. 11–38). Chicago: University of Chicago Press.

Haith, M. M. (1997, April). *Who put the "cog" in infant cognition? Is rich interpretation too costly?* Paper presented at the meeting of the Society for Research in Child Development, Washington, DC.

Haith, M. M., Benson, J. B., Roberts, R. J., & Pennington, B. F. (1994). *The development of future-oriented processes.* Chicago: University of Chicago Press.

Haith, M. M., Hazen, C., & Goodman, G. S. (1988). Expectation and anticipation of dynamic visual events by 3.5-month-old babies. *Child Development, 59,* 467–479.

Halbwachs, M. (1980). *Collective memory.* New York: Harper & Row.

Hamond, N. R., & Fivush, R. (1991). Memories of Mickey Mouse: Young children recount their trip to Disneyworld. *Cognitive Development, 6,* 433–448.

Harley, K., & Reese, E. (1999). Origins of autobiographical memory. *Developmental Psychology, 35,* 1338–1348.

Harre, R. (1984). *Personal being: A theory for individual psychology.* Cambridge, MA: Harvard University Press.

Hartup, W. (1985). Relationships and their significance in cognitive development. In R. Hinde & A. Perret-Clermont (Eds.), *Relationships and cognitive development* (pp. 66–82). Oxford, UK: Oxford University Press.

Hatano, G., Miyake, Y., & Binks, M. (1977). Performance of expert abacus operators. *Cognition, 9,* 47–55.

Hawkins, J., Homolsky, M., & Heide, P. (1984). *Paired problem solving in a computer context* (Technical Report No. 33). New York: Bank Street College of Education.

Hayes-Roth, B. (1980). *Estimation of time requirements during planning: Interactions between motivation and cognition* (Rand Note: N-1581-ONR). Santa Monica, CA: Rand Corporation.

Heath, S. B. (1983). *Ways with words: Language, life, and work in communities and classrooms.* Cambridge, UK: Cambridge University Press.

Hirschberg, L. M., & Svejda, M. (1990). When infants look to their parents: 1. Infants' social referencing of mothers compared to fathers. *Child Development, 61,* 1175–1186.

Hirst, W., & Manier, D. (1996). Remembering as communication: A family recounts its past. In D. Rubin (Ed.), *Remembering our past: Studies in autobiographical memory* (pp. 271–290). New York: Cambridge University Press.

Howe, M. L., & Courage, M. L. (1993). On resolving the enigma of infantile amnesia. *Psychological Bulletin, 113,* 305–326.

Howe, M. L., Courage, M. L., & Peterson, C. (1994). How can I remember when

"I" wasn't there: Long-term retention of traumatic experiences and the emergence of the cognitive self. *Consciousness and Cognition, 3*, 327–355.

Hudson, J. A. (1990). The emergence of autobiographical memory in mother–child conversation. In R. Fivush & J. A. Hudson (Eds.), *Knowing and remembering in young children* (pp. 166–196). Cambridge, UK: Cambridge University Press.

Hudson, J. A. (1991). Learning to reminisce: A case study. *Journal of Narrative and Life History, 1*, 295–324.

Hudson, J. A., & Fivush, R. (1990). Introduction: What young children remember and why. In R. Fivush & J. A. Hudson (Eds.), *Knowing and remembering in young children* (pp. 1–8). Cambridge, UK: Cambridge University Press.

Hudson, J. A., & Fivush, R. (1991). Planning in the preschool years: The emergence of plans from general event knowledge. *Cognitive Development, 6*, 393–415.

Itard, J. M. G. (1982). *The wild boy of Aveyron*. New York: Appleton-Century-Crofts. (Original work published 1801)

Johnson, M. (1997). *Developmental cognitive neuroscience*. Cambridge, MA: Blackwell.

Kail, R. (1991). Developmental change in speed of processing during childhood and adolescence. *Developmental Psychology, 109*, 490–501.

Karmiloff-Smith, A. (1995). *Beyond modularity: A developmental perspective on cognitive science*. Cambridge, MA: MIT Press.

Kearins, J. M. (1981). Visual spatial memory in Australian aboriginal children of desert regions. *Cognitive Psychology, 13*, 434–460.

Klahr, D. (1982). Non-monotone assessment of monotone development: An information processing analysis. In S. Strauss &. R. Stavy (Eds.), *U-shaped behavioral growth* (pp. 63–86). New York: Academic Press.

Klahr, D. (1992). Information processing approaches to cognitive development. In M. H. Bornstein & M. E. Lamb (Eds.), *Developmental psychology: An advanced textbook* (3rd ed., pp. 273–335). Hillsdale, NJ: Erlbaum.

Klahr, D., & Robinson, M. (1981). Formal assessment of problem solving and planning processes in preschool children. *Cognitive Psychology, 13*, 113–148.

Klahr, D., & Wallace, J. G. (1976). *Cognitive development: An information processing view*. Hillsdale, NJ: Erlbaum.

Klinnert, M. D. (1984). The regulation of infant behavior by maternal facial expression. *Infant Behavior and Development, 7*, 447–465.

Klinnert, M. D., Emde, R. N., Butterfield, P., & Campos, J. J. (1986). Social referencing: The infant's use of emotional signals from a friendly adult with mother present. *Developmental Psychology, 22*, 427–434.

Kopp, C. B. (1997). Young children's emotion management, instrumental control, and plans. In S. L. Friedman & E. K. Scholnick (Eds.), *The developmental psychology of planning: Why, how, and when do we plan?* (pp. 103–124). Hillsdale, NJ: Erlbaum.

Kopp, C. B., & Vaughn, B. E. (1982). Sustained attention during exploratory manipulation as a predictor of cognitive competence in preterm infants. *Child Development, 53*, 174–182.

Krietler, S., & Krietler, H. (1987). Conceptions and processes of planning: The developmental perspective. In S. Friedman, E. Scholnick, & R. R. Cocking (Eds.), *Blueprints for thinking: The role of planning in cognitive development* (pp. 205–272). Cambridge, UK: Cambridge University Press.

Kruger, A. C. (1992). The effect of peer and adult–child transactive discussions on moral reasoning. *Merrill–Palmer Quarterly, 38*, 191–211.

Kuhn, D., Garcia-Mila, M., Zohar, Z., & Andersen, C. (1995). Strategies of knowledge acquisition. *Monographs of the Society for Research in Child Development, 60*(4, Serial No. 245), 1–127.

Kurtz, B. E., Schneider, W., Carr, M., Borkowski, J. G., & Rellinger, E. (1990). Strategy instruction and attributional beliefs in West Germany and the United States: Do teachers foster metacognitive development? *Contemporary Educational Psychology, 15*, 268–283.

Laasko, M. L. (1995). Mothers' and fathers' communication clarity and teaching strategies with their school-age children. *Journal of Applied Developmental Psychology, 16*, 445–461.

Laosa, L. M. (1980). Maternal teaching strategies in Chicano and Anglo-American families: The influence of culture and education on maternal behavior. *Child Development, 51*, 759–765.

Lave, J., & Wenger, E. (1991). *Situated learning: Legitimate peripheral participation.* Cambridge, UK: Cambridge University Press.

Leont'ev, A. N. (1981). The problem of activity in psychology. In J. V. Wertsch (Ed.), *The concept of activity in Soviet psychology* (pp. 37–71). Armonk, NY: M. E. Sharpe.

Levinson, S. C. (1996). Frames of reference and Molyneux's question: Cross-linguistic evidence. In P. Bloom, M. A. Peterson, L. Nadel, & M. F. Garrett (Eds.), *Language and space* (pp. 109–169). Cambridge, MA: MIT Press.

Levy, E., & Nelson, K. (1994). Words in discourse: A dialectical approach to the acquisition of meaning and use. *Journal of Child Language, 21*, 367–389.

Lewin, K. (1964). *Field theory in social science.* New York: Harper.

Lewis, M., & Brooks-Gunn, J. (1979). *Social cognition and the acquisition of the self.* New York: Plenum Press.

Lucariello, J., & Nelson, K. (1987). Remembering and planning talk between mothers and children. *Discourse Processes, 10*, 219–235.

Luria, A. R. (1961). *The role of speech in the regulation of normal and abnormal behavior.* New York: Liveright.

Luria, A. R. (1976). *Cognitive development: Its cultural and social foundations.* Cambridge, MA: Harvard University Press.

Maccoby, E. E. (1994). The role of parents in the socialization of children: An historical overview. In R. D. Parke, P. A. Ornstein, J. J. Rieser, & C. Zahn-Waxler (Eds.), *A century of developmental psychology* (pp. 589–615). Washington, DC: American Psychological Association.

Mackie, D. (1980). A cross-cultural study of intra- and interindividual conflicts of centrations. *European Journal of Social Psychology, 10*, 313–318.

Mackie, D. (1983). The effect of social interaction on conservation of spatial relations. *Journal of Cross-Cultural Psychology, 14*, 131–151.

Macfarlane, J. A. (1975). Olfaction in the development of social preferences in the human neonate. In M. A. Hofer (Ed.), *Parent–infant interaction* (pp. 103–117). Amsterdam: Elsevier.

MacWhinney, B. (1987). *Mechanisms of language acquisition.* Hillsdale, NJ: Erlbaum.

Mandler, J. (1984). *Stories, scripts, and scenes: Aspects of schema theory.* Hillsdale, NJ: Erlbaum.

Martini, M., & Kirkpatrick, J. (1981). Early interactions in the Marquesas Islands. In T. M. Fields, A. M. Sostek, P. Vietze, & P. H. Leiderman (Eds.), *Culture and early interactions* (pp. 189–213). Hillsdale, NJ: Erlbaum.

Matas, L., Arend, R. A., & Sroufe, L. A. (1978). Continuity of adaptation in the second year: The relationship between quality of attachment and later competence. *Child Development, 49,* 547–556.

Mayes, F. (1996). *Under the Tuscan sun.* San Francisco: Chronicle Books.

McLane, J. B. (1981). *Dyadic problem solving: A comparison of child–child and mother–child interaction.* Unpublished doctoral dissertation, Northwestern University, Evanston, IL.

Mead, M. (1935). *Sex and temperament in three primitive societies.* New York: Morrow.

Mead, M. (1949). *Male and female.* New York: Morrow.

Mead, M. (1972). *Blackberry winter: My earlier years.* New York: Kodansha International.

Middleton, D. (1997). The social organization of conversational remembering: Experience as individual and collective concerns. *Mind, Culture, and Activity, 4,* 71–85.

Miller, G. A. (1956). The magical number seven, plus or minus two: Some limits on our capacity for processing information. *Psychological Review, 63,* 81–97.

Miller, P. H. (1990). The development of strategies of selective attention. In D. F. Bjorkland (Ed.), *Children's strategies: Contemporary views of cognitive development* (pp. 157–184). Hillsdale, NJ: Erlbaum.

Miller, P. H. (1993). *Theories of developmental psychology* (3rd ed.). New York: Freeman.

Miller, P. H., Woody-Ramsey, J., & Aloise, P. A. (1991). The role of strategy effortfulness in strategy effectiveness. *Developmental Psychology, 27,* 738–745.

Miller, P. J., & Moore, B. B. (1989). Narrative conjunctions of caregiver and child: A comparative perspective on socialization through stories. *Ethos, 17,* 428–449.

Miller, P. J., & Sperry, L. L. (1988). Early talk about the past: The origins of conversational stories of personal experience. *Journal of Child Language, 15,* 293–315.

Mistry, J. (1997). The development of remembering in cultural context. In N. Cowan (Ed.), *The development of memory in childhood* (pp. 343–368). Hove, East Sussex, UK: Psychology Press.

Morelli, G. A., Rogoff, B., & Angelillo, C. (1993, April). *Cultural variation in children's work and social activities.* Paper presented at the meeting of the Society for Research in Child Development, New Orleans, LA.

Moss, E. (1992). The socioaffective context of joint cognitive activity. In L. T. Winegar & J. Valsiner (Eds.), *Children's development within social context: Vol. 2. Research and methodology* (pp. 117–154). Hillsdale, NJ: Erlbaum.

Mullen, M. K., & Yi, S. (1995). The cultural context of talk about the past: Implications for the development of autobiographical memory. *Cognitive Development, 10*, 407–419.

Munroe, R. L., & Munroe, R. H. (1971). Effect of environmental experience on spatial ability in an East African society. *Journal of Social Psychology, 83*, 155–185.

Murray, L., & Trevarthen, C. (1985). Emotional regulation of interactions between two-month-olds and their mothers. In T. M. Field & N. A. Fox (Eds.), *Social perception in infants* (pp. 177–197). Norwood, NJ: Ablex.

Naus, M. J., & Ornstein, P. A. (1983). Development of memory strategies: Analysis, questions, and issues. In M.T.H. Chi (Ed.), *Trends in memory development research* (pp. 1–29). New York: Karger.

Neisser, U. (1982). *Memory observed: Remembering in natural contexts.* New York: Freeman.

Nelson, K. (1989). *Narratives from the crib.* Cambridge, MA: Harvard University Press.

Nelson, K. (1990). Remembering, forgetting, and childhood amnesia. In R. Fivush & J. Hudson (Eds.), *Knowing and remembering in young children* (pp. 301–316). Cambridge, UK: Cambridge University Press.

Nelson, K. (1993). The psychological and social origins of autobiographical memory. *Psychological Science, 4*, 7–14.

Nelson, K. (1996). *Language in cognitive development.* Cambridge, UK: Cambridge University Press.

Nelson, K., & Gruendel, J. (1981). Generalized event representations: Basic building blocks of cognitive development. In M. E. Lamb & A. L. Brown (Eds.), *Advances in developmental psychology* (Vol. 1, pp. 131–158). Hillsdale, NJ: Erlbaum.

Nerlove, S. B., & Snipper, A. S. (1981). Cognitive consequences of cultural opportunity. In R. H. Munroe, R. L. Munroe, & B. B. Whiting (Eds.), *Handbook of cross-cultural human development* (pp. 423–474). New York: Garland.

Newport, E., Gleitman, L., & Gleitman, H. (1977). "Mother I'd rather do it myself": Some effects and non-effects of maternal speech style. In C. E. Snow & C. A. Ferguson (Eds.), *Talking to children: Language input and acquisition* (pp. 126–165). Cambridge, UK: Cambridge University Press.

Ninio, A., & Bruner, J. S. (1978). Achievement and antecedents of labeling. *Journal of Child Language, 5*, 11–15.

Pacifici, C., & Bearison, D. J. (1991). Development of children's self-regulations in idealized and mother–child interactions. *Cognitive Development, 6*, 261–277.

Palinscar, A. S., & Brown, A. L. (1984). Reciprocal teaching of comprehension-monitoring activities. *Cognition and Instruction, 1*, 117–175.

Palinscar, A. S., Brown, A. L., & Campione, J. C. (1993). First-grade dialogues for knowledge acquisition and use. In E. A. Forman, N. Minick, & C. A. Stone (Eds.), *Contexts for learning: Sociocultural dynamics in children's development* (pp. 43–57). New York: Oxford University Press.

Parinello, R. M., & Ruff, H. A. (1988). The influence of adult intervention on infants' level of attention. *Child Development, 59*, 1125–1135.

Parke, R. D. (1996). *Fatherhood.* Cambridge, MA: Cambridge University Press.

Parke, R. D., & Bhavnagri, N. P. (1989). Parents as managers of children's peer relationships. In D. Belle (Ed.), *Children's social networks and social supports* (pp. 241–259). New York: Wiley.

Parke, R. D., & Buriel, R. (1998). Socialization in the family: Ethnic and ecological perspectives. In W. Damon (Series Ed.) & N. Eisenberg (Vol. Ed.), *Handbook of child psychology: Vol. 3. Social, emotional, and personality development* (pp. 463–552). New York: Wiley.

Parrila, R. K., Aysto, S., & Das, J. P. (1994). Development of planning in relation to age, attention, simultaneous and successive processing. *Journal of Psychoeducational Assessment, 12*, 212–227.

Pascual-Leone, J. A. (1970). A mathematical model for transition in Piaget's developmental stages. *Acta Psychologica, 32*, 301–345.

Pea, R. D. (1982). What is planning the development of? In D. L. Forbes & M. T. Greenberg (Eds.), *Children's planning strategies* (pp. 5–27). San Francisco: Jossey-Bass.

Pea, R. D., & Hawkins, J. (1987). Children's planning processes in a chore-scheduling task. In S. L. Friedman, E. K. Scholnick, & R. R. Cocking (Eds.), *Blueprints for thinking: The role of planning in psychological development* (pp. 273–302). Cambridge, UK: Cambridge University Press.

Penner, D. E., & Klahr, D. (1996). The interaction of domain-specific knowledge and domain-general discovery strategies: A study with sinking objects. *Child Development, 67*, 2709–2727.

Perez-Granados, D. R., & Callanan, M. A. (1997). Conversations with mothers and siblings: Young children's semantic and conceptual development. *Developmental Psychology, 33*, 120–134.

Piaget, J. (1926). *The language and thought of the child.* New York: Harcourt, Brace.

Piaget, J., & Inhelder, B. (1956). *The child's conception of space.* New York: Norton.

Pine, K. J., & Messer, D. J. (1998). Group collaboration effects and the explicitness of children's knowledge. *Cognitive Development, 13*, 109–126.

Plomin, R. (1990). *Nature and nurture: An introduction to behavioral genetics.* Belmont, CA: Brooks/Cole.

Plumert, J. M., & Nichols-Whitehead, P. (1996). Parental scaffolding of young children's spatial communication. *Developmental Psychology, 32*, 523–532.

Porges, S. W. (1983). Heart rate patterns in neonates: A potential diagnostic window to the brain. In T. Field & A. Sostek (Eds.), *Infants born at risk: Physiological, perceptual, and cognitive processes* (pp. 3–22). New York: Grune & Stratton.

Pratt, M. W., Kerig, P., Cowan, P. A., & Cowan, C. P. (1988). Mothers and fathers teaching 3-year-olds: Authoritative parenting and adult scaffolding of young children's learning. *Development Psychology, 24*, 832–839.

Pressley, M., Borkowski, J. G., & Schneider, W. (1987). Cognitive strategies: Good strategy users coordinate metacognition and knowledge. In R. Vasta (Ed.), *Annals of child development* (Vol. 4, pp. 89–129). Greenwich, CT: JAI Press.

Presson, C. C. (1987). The development of spatial cognition: Secondary uses of spatial information. In N. Eisenberg (Ed.), *Contemporary topics in developmental psychology* (pp. 77–112). New York: Wiley.

Pribram, K. H., & Luria, A. R. (1973). *Psychophysiology of the frontal lobes.* New York: Academic Press.

Radziszewska, B., & Rogoff, B. (1988). Influence of adult and peer collaborators on children's planning skills. *Developmental Psychology, 24,* 840–848.

Radziszewska, B., & Rogoff, B. (1991). Children's guided participation in planning imaginary errands with skilled adult or peer partners. *Developmental Psychology, 27,* 381–389.

Ratner, H. H. (1980). The role of social context in memory development. In M. Perlmutter (Ed.), *Children's memory* (pp. 49–67). San Francisco: Jossey-Bass.

Ratner, H. H. (1984). Memory demands and the development of young children's memory. *Child Development, 55,* 2173–2191.

Reese, E., & Fivush, R. (1993). Parental styles of talking about the past. *Developmental Psychology, 29,* 596–606.

Reese, E., Haden, C. A., & Fivush, R. (1993). Mother–child conversations about the past: Relationships of style and memory over time. *Cognitive Development, 8,* 403–430.

Reiss, D. (1981). *The family's construction of reality.* Cambridge, MA: Harvard University Press.

Renshaw, P. D., & Gardner, R. (1990). Process versus product task interpretation and parental teaching practices. *International Journal of Behavioral Development, 13,* 489–505.

Repacholi, B. M. (1998). Infants' use of attentional cues to identify the referent of another person's emotional expression. *Developmental Psychology, 34,* 1017–1025.

Reznick, J. S. (1994). In search of infant expectation. In M. M. Haith, J. B. Benson, R. J. Roberts, & B. F. Pennington (Eds.), *The development of future-oriented processes* (pp. 39–59). Chicago: University of Chicago Press.

Ridderinkhof, K. R., & van der Molen, M. (1995). A psychophysiological analysis of developmental differences in the ability to resist interference. *Child Development, 60,* 1040–1056.

Riegel, K. F. (1979). *Foundations of a dialectical psychology.* New York: Academic Press.

Rodriguez, R. (1982). *Hunger of memory: The education of Richard Rodriguez.* New York: Bantam Books.

Rogoff, B. (1981). Schooling and the development of cognitive skills. In H. C. Triandis & A. Heron (Eds.), *Handbook of cross-cultural psychology* (Vol. 4, pp. 233–294). Rockleigh, NJ: Allyn & Bacon.

Rogoff, B. (1990). *Apprenticeship in thinking: Cognitive development in social context.* New York: Oxford University Press.

Rogoff, B. (1996). Developmental transitions in children's participation in sociocultural activities. In A. J. Sameroff & M. M. Haith (Eds.), *The five to seven year shift: The age of reason and responsibility* (pp. 273–294). Chicago: University of Chicago Press.

Rogoff, B. (1998). Cognition as a collaborative process. In W. Damon (Series Ed.) & D. Kuhn & R. S. Siegler (Vol. Eds.), *Handbook of child psychology: Cognition, perception, and language* (pp. 679–744). New York: Wiley.

Rogoff, B., Ellis, S., & Gardner, W. (1984). The adjustment of adult–child instruction according to child's age and task. *Developmental Psychology, 20,* 193–199.

Rogoff, B., & Gardner, W. P. (1984). Adult guidance of cognitive development. In B. Rogoff & J. Lave (Eds.), *Everyday cognition: Its development in social context* (pp. 95–116). Harvard, MA: Cambridge University Press.

Rogoff, B., & Gauvain, M. (1986). A method for the analysis of patterns, illustrated with data on mother–child instructional interaction. In J. Valsiner (Ed.), *The role of the individual subject in scientific psychology* (pp. 261–290). New York: Plenum Press.

Rogoff, B., Gauvain, M., & Ellis, S. (1984). Development viewed in its cultural context. In M. H. Bornstein & M. E. Lamb (Eds.), *Developmental psychology* (pp. 533–571). Hillsdale, NJ: Erlbaum.

Rogoff, B., Gauvain, M., & Gardner, W. P. (1987). The development of children's skill at adjusting plans to circumstances. In S. L. Friedman, E. K. Scholnick, & R. R. Cocking (Eds.), *Blueprints for thinking: The role of planning in cognitive development* (pp. 303–320). Cambridge, UK: Cambridge University Press.

Rogoff, B., Malkin, C., & Gilbride, K. (1984). Interaction with babies as guidance in cognitive development. In B. Rogoff & J. V. Wertsch (Eds.), *Children's learning in the "zone of proximal development"* (pp. 31–44). San Francisco: Jossey-Bass.

Rogoff, B., & Mistry, J. (1985). The social and functional context of children's remembering. In R. Fivush & J. A. Hudson (Eds.), *Knowing and remembering in young children* (pp. 197–222). Cambridge, UK: Cambridge University Press.

Rogoff, B., Mistry, J., Radziszewska, & Germond, J. (1992). Infants' instrumental social interaction with adults. In S. Feinman (Ed.), *Social referencing and the social construction of reality in infancy* (pp. 297–348). New York: Plenum Press.

Rogoff, B., & Waddell, K. J. (1982). Memory for information organized in a scene by children from two cultures. *Child Development, 53*, 1224–1228.

Rogoff, B., & Wertsch, J. V. (Eds.). (1984). *Children's learning in the "zone of proximal development."* San Francisco: Jossey-Bass.

Rommetveit, R. (1974). *On message structure: A framework for the study of language and communication.* London: Wiley.

Rommetveit, R. (1985). Language acquisition as increasing linguistic structuring of experience and symbolic behavior control. In J. V. Wertsch (Ed.), *Culture, communication, and cognition: Vygotskian perspectives* (pp. 183–204). Cambridge, UK: Cambridge University Press.

Roosevelt, E. (1961). *The autobiography of Eleanor Roosevelt.* New York: De Capo Press.

Rosen, W. D., Adamson, L. B., & Bakeman, R. (1992). An experimental investigation of infant social referencing: Mothers' messages and gender differences. *Developmental Psychology, 28*, 1172–1178.

Rosenshine, B., & Meister, C. (1994). Reciprocal teaching: A review of research. *Review of Educational Research, 64*, 479–530.

Roth, C. (1983). Factors affecting developmental changes in the speed of processing. *Journal of Experimental Child Psychology, 35*, 509–528.

Rothbart, M. K., & Bates, J. E. (1998). Temperament. In W. Damon (Series Ed.) & N. Eisenberg (Vol. Ed.), *Handbook of child psychology: Vol. 3. Social, emotional, and personality development* (pp. 105–176). New York: Wiley.

Ruble, D. N., Boggiano, A. K., Feldman, N. S., & Loebl, J. H. (1980). A developmental analysis of the role of social comparison in self-evaluation. *Developmental Psychology, 16,* 105–115.

Ruble, D. N., & Frey, K. S. (1987). Social comparison and self-evaluation in the classroom: Developmental changes in knowledge and function. In J. C. Masters & W. P. Smith (Eds.), *Social comparison, social justice, and relative deprivation: Theoretical, empirical, and policy perspectives* (pp. 84–104). Hillsdale, NJ: Erlbaum.

Ruff, H. A., & Rothbart, M. K. (1996). *Attention in early development: Themes and variations.* New York: Oxford University Press.

Saarni, C., Mumme, D., & Campos, J. J. (1998). Emotional development: Action, communication, and understanding. In W. Damon (Series Ed.) & N. Eisenberg (Vol. Ed.), *Handbook of child psychology: Vol. 3. Social, emotional, and personality development* (pp. 237–309). New York: Wiley.

Sahlins, M. D. (1976). *Culture and practical reason.* Chicago: University of Chicago Press.

Sameroff, A. J., & Haith, M. M. (Eds.). (1996). *The five to seven year shift: The age of reason and responsibility.* Chicago: University of Chicago Press.

Samuel, J., & Bryant, P. (1984). Asking only one question in the conservation experiment. *Journal of Child Psychology and Psychiatry, 25,* 315–318.

Saxe, G. B. (1991). *Culture and cognitive development: Studies in mathematical understanding.* Hillsdale, NJ: Erlbaum.

Saxe, G. B., Guberman, S. R., & Gearhart, M. (1987). Social processes in early number development. *Monographs of the Society for Research in Child Development, 52*(2, Serial No. 216), 3–162.

Scaife, M., & Bruner, J. S. (1975). The capacity for joint visual attention in the infant. *Nature, 253,* 265–266.

Schaffer, H. R. (1977). *Studies in mother–infant interaction.* London: Academic Press.

Schaffer, H. R. (1992). Joint involvement episodes as contexts for cognitive development. In H. McGurk (Ed.), *Childhood social development: Contemporary perspectives* (pp. 99–129). Hove, Sussex, UK: Erlbaum.

Schiff, A. R., & Knopf, I. J. (1985). The effect of task demands on attention allocation in children of different ages. *Child Development, 56,* 621–630.

Schneider, W., & Bjorkland, D. F. (1998). Memory. In W. Damon (Series Ed.) & D. Kuhn & R. S. Siegler (Vol. Eds.), *Handbook of child psychology: Cognition, perception, and language* (pp. 467–521). New York: Wiley.

Schneider, W., & Pressley, M. (1989). *Memory development between 2 and 20* (1st ed.). New York: Springer.

Schneider, W., & Pressley, M. (1997). *Memory development between 2 and 20* (2nd ed.). Mahwah, NJ: Erlbaum.

Scribner, S. (1985). Vygotsky's use of history. In J. V. Wertsch (Ed.), *Culture, communication, and cognition: Vygotskian perspectives* (pp. 119–145). Cambridge, UK: Cambridge University Press.

Selman, R. L. (1980). *The growth of interpersonal understanding.* New York: Academic Press.

Shotter, J. (1990). The social construction of forgetting and remembering. In D. Middleton & D. Edwards (Eds.), *Collective memory* (pp. 120–138). London: Sage.

Siegel, M. (1991). *Knowing children: Experiments in conversation and cognition*. London: Erlbaum.

Siegler, R. S. (1976). Three aspects of cognitive development. *Cognitive Psychology, 8,* 481–520.

Siegler, R. S. (1989). Mechanisms of cognitive development. *American Review of Psychology, 40,* 353–379.

Siegler, R. S. (1996). *Emerging minds: The process of change in children's thinking*. New York: Oxford University Press.

Siegler, R. S. (1998). *Children's thinking* (3rd ed.). Upper Saddle River, NJ: Prentice-Hall.

Sigel, I. E. (1970). The distancing hypothesis: A causal hypothesis for the acquisition of representational thought. In M. R. Jones (Ed.), *Miami Symposium on the Prediction of Behavior: Effect of early experience* (pp. 99–118). Coral Gables, FL: University of Miami Press.

Sigman, M., & Kasari, C. (1995). Joint attention across contexts in normal and autistic children. In C. Moore & P. J. Dunham (Eds.), *Joint attention: Its origins and role in development* (pp. 189–203). Hillsdale, NJ: Erlbaum.

Snow, C. E. (1990). Building memories: The ontogeny of autobiography. In D. Cicchetti & M. Beeghly (Eds.), *The self in transition: Infancy to childhood* (pp. 213–242). Chicago: University of Chicago Press.

Soyinka, W. (1981). *Aké: The years of childhood*. New York: Vantage Books.

Stern, D. N. (1977). *The first relationship: Mother and infant*. Cambridge, MA: Harvard University Press.

Stern, D. N. (1985). *The interpersonal world of the infant: A view from psychoanalysis and developmental psychology*. New York: Basic Books.

Sternberg, R. J. (1984). *Mechanisms of cognitive development*. New York: Freeman.

Sternberg, R. J. (1985). *Beyond IQ: A triadic theory of human intelligence*. New York: Cambridge University Press.

Sternberg, R. J., & Wagner, R. (1986). *Practical intelligence*. Cambridge, UK: Cambridge University Press.

Stevenson, H. W. (1982). Influences of schooling on cognitive development. In D. A. Wagner & H. W. Stevenson (Eds.), *Cultural perspectives on child development* (pp. 208–224). San Francisco: Freeman.

Stevenson, H. W., & Stigler, J. W. (1992). *The learning gap: Why our schools are failing and what we can learn from Japanese and Chinese education*. New York: Summit Books.

Stigler, J. W. (1984). Mental abacus: The effect of abacus training on Chinese children's mental calculations. *Cognitive Psychology, 16,* 145–176.

Stigler, J. W., Chalip, L., & Miller, K. F. (1986). Consequences of skill: The case of abacus training in Taiwan. *American Journal of Education, 94,* 447–479.

Super, C. M., & Harkness, S. (1986). The developmental niche: A conceptualization at the interface of child and culture. *International Journal of Behavioral Development, 9,* 545–569.

Swetz, F. J. (1987). *Capitalism and arithmetic*. LaSalle, IL: Open Court.

Tamis-LaMonda, C. S., & Bornstein, M. H. (1989). Habituation and maternal encouragement of attention in infancy as predictors of toddler language, play, and representational competence. *Child Development, 60,* 738–751.

Teasley, S. D. (1995). The role of talk in children's peer collaboration. *Developmental Psychology, 31*, 207–220.

Tessler, M., & Nelson, K. (1994). Making memories: The influence of joint encoding on later recall. *Consciousness and Cognition, 3*, 307–326.

Thompson, R. (1998). Early sociopersonality development. In W. Damon (Series Ed.) & N. Eisenberg (Vol. Ed.), *Handbook of child psychology: Social, emotional, and personality development* (pp. 25–104). New York: Wiley.

Tomasello, M. (1988). The role of joint attentional processes in early language development. *Language Sciences, 10*, 69–88.

Tomasello, M. (1995). Joint attention as social cognition. In C. Moore & P. H. Dunham (Eds.), *Joint attention: Its origins and role in development* (pp. 103–130). Hillsdale, NJ: Erlbaum.

Tomasello, M., Conti-Ramsden, G., & Ewert, B. (1990). Young children's conversations with their mothers and fathers: Differences in breakdown and repair. *Journal of Child Language, 17*, 115–130.

Tomasello, M., & Farrar, M. J. (1986). Joint attention and early language. *Child Development, 57*, 1454–1463.

Trevarthen, C. (1980a). The foundations of intersubjectivity: Development of interpersonal and cooperative understanding in infants. In D. R. Olson (Ed.), *The social foundations of language and thought* (pp. 316–342). New York: Norton.

Trevarthen, C. (1980b). Instincts for human understanding and for cultural co-operation: Their development in infancy. In M. von Cranach, K. Foppa, W. Lepenies, & D. Ploog (Eds.), *Human ethology: Claims and limits of a new discipline* (pp. 530–594). Cambridge, UK: Cambridge University Press.

Trevarthen, C. (1988). Universal co-operative motives: How infants begin to know the language and culture of their parents. In G. Jahoda & I. M. Lewis (Eds.), *Acquiring culture: Cross cultural studies in child development* (pp. 37–90). London: Croom Helm.

Tudge, J. R. H., & Rogoff, B. (1989). Peer influences on cognitive development: Piagetian and Vygotskian perspectives. In M. Bornstein & J. Bruner (Eds.), *Interaction in human development* (pp. 17–40). Hillsdale, NJ: Erlbaum.

Tulving, E. (1983). *Elements of episodic memory.* New York: Oxford University Press.

Valsiner, J. (1984). Construction in the zone of proximal development in adult–child joint action: The socialization of meals. In B. Rogoff & J. V. Wertsch (Eds.), *Children's learning in the "zone of proximal development"* (pp. 65–76). San Francisco: Jossey-Bass.

Valsiner, J. (1989). *Human development and culture: The social nature of personality and its study.* Lexington, MA: Lexington Books.

Von Hofsten, C. (1994). Planning and perceiving what is going to happen next. In M. M. Haith, J. B. Benson, R. J. Roberts, & B. F. Pennington (Eds.), *The development of future-oriented processes* (pp. 63–86). Chicago: University of Chicago Press.

Vurpillot, E. (1968). The development of scanning strategies and their relation to visual differentiation. *Journal of Experimental Child Psychology, 6*, 632–650.

Vygotsky, L. S. (1962). *Thought and language.* New York: Wiley.

Vygotsky, L. S. (1978). *Mind in society: The development of higher mental functions.* Cambridge, MA: Harvard University Press.

Vygotsky, L. S. (1981). The genesis of higher mental functions. In J. V. Wertsch (Ed.), *The concept of activity in Soviet psychology* (pp. 144–188). Armonk, NY: M. E. Sharpe.

Vygotsky, L. S. (1986). *Thought and language.* Cambridge, MA: MIT Press.

Vygotsky, L. S. (1987). *The collected works of L. S. Vygotsky: Vol. 1. Problems of general psychology.* New York: Plenum Press.

Walden, T., & Ogan, T. (1988). Development of social referencing. *Child Development, 59,* 1230–1240.

Walker-Andrews, A. S. (1997). Infants' perceptions of expressive behaviors: Differentiation of multimodal information. *Psychological Bulletin, 121,* 437–456.

Weisner, T. S. (1996). The 5 to 7 transition as an ecocultural project. In A. J. Sameroff & M. M. Haith (Eds.), *The five to seven year shift: The age of reason and responsibility* (pp. 295–326). Chicago: University of Chicago Press.

Weiss, M.J.S., & Zelazo, P. R. (1991). *Newborn attention: Biological constraints and the influence of experience.* Norwood, NJ: Ablex.

Welch-Ross, M. K. (1997). Mother–child participation in conversation about the past: Relationship to preschoolers' theory of mind. *Developmental Psychology, 33,* 618–629.

Weldon, M. S., & Bellinger, K. D. (1997). Collective memory: Collaborative and individual processes in remembering. *Journal of Experimental Psychology: Learning, Memory, and Cognition, 23,* 1160–1175.

Wellman, H. M., Fabricius, W. V., & Sophian, C. (1985). The early development of planning. In H. M. Wellman (Ed.), *Children's searching: The development of search skill and spatial representation* (pp. 123–150). Hillsdale, NJ: Erlbaum.

Wertsch, J. V. (1978). Adult–child interaction and the roots of metacognition. *Quarterly Newsletter of the Institute for Comparative Human Development, 2,* 15–18.

Wertsch, J. V. (Ed.). (1981). *The concept of activity in Soviet psychology.* Armonk, NY: M. E. Sharpe.

Wertsch, J. V. (1985). *Vygotsky and the social formation of mind.* Cambridge, MA: Harvard University Press.

Wertsch, J. V., del Rio, P., & Alvarez, A. (Eds.). (1995). *Sociocultural studies of mind.* Cambridge, UK: Cambridge University Press.

Wertsch, J. V., McNamee, G. D., McLane, J. B., & Budwig, N. A. (1980). The adult–child dyad as a problem-solving system. *Child Development, 51,* 1215–1221.

Wertsch, J. V., Minick, N., & Arns, F. J. (1984). The creation of context in joint problem solving. In B. Rogoff & J. Lave (Eds.), *Everyday cognition: Its development in social context* (pp. 151–171). Cambridge, MA: Harvard University Press.

Wertsch, J. V., & Tulviste, P. (1994). Lev Semyonovich Vygotsky and contemporary developmental psychology. In R. D. Parke, P. A. Ornstein, J. J. Rieser, & C. Zahn-Waxler (Eds.), *A century of developmental psychology* (pp. 333–355). Washington, DC: American Psychological Association.

White, S. J., & Siegel, A. W. (1984). Cognitive development in time and space. In B. Rogoff & J. Lave (Eds.), *Everyday cognition: Its development in social context* (pp. 238–277). Cambridge, MA: Harvard University Press.

Whiting, B. B. (1980). Culture and social behavior: A model for the development of social behavior. *Ethos, 8*, 95–116.

Whiting, B. B., & Edwards, C. P. (1988). *Children of different worlds: The formation of social behavior.* Cambridge, MA: Harvard University Press.

Willatts, P. (1990). Development of problem solving strategies in infants. In D. F. Bjorkland (Ed.), *Children's strategies* (pp. 23–66). Hillsdale, NJ: Erlbaum.

Wood, D. J., Bruner, J. S., & Ross, G. (1976). The role of tutoring in problem-solving. *Journal of Child Psychology and Psychiatry, 17*, 89–100.

Wood, D. J., & Middleton, D. (1975). A study of assisted problem solving. *British Journal of Psychology, 66*, 181–191.

Wood, D. J., Wood, H., & Middleton, D. (1978). An experimental evaluation of four face-to-face teaching strategies. *International Journal of Behavioral Development, 2*, 131–147.

Worden, P. E., Kee, D. W., & Ingle, M. J. (1987). Parental teaching strategies with preschoolers: A comparison of mothers and fathers within different alphabet tasks. *Contemporary Educational Psychology, 12*, 95–109.

Zajonc, R. B., & Markus, H. (1985). Affect and cognition: The hard interface. In C. E. Izard, J. Kagan, & R. Zajonc (Eds.), *Emotions, cognition, and behavior* (pp. 73–102). New York: Cambridge University Press.

Zarbatany, L., & Lamb, M. E. (1985). Social referencing as a function of information source: Mothers versus strangers. *Infant Behavior and Development, 8*, 25–33.

Zinchenko, P. I. (1981). Involuntary memory and the goal-directed nature of activity in Soviet psychology. In J. V. Wertsch (Ed.), *The concept of activity in Soviet psychology* (pp. 300–340). Armonk, NY: M. E. Sharpe.

Zinchenko, V. P. (1995). Cultural–historical psychology and the psychological theory of activity: Retrospect and prospect. In J. V. Wertsch, P. del Rio, & A. Alvarez (Eds.), *Sociocultural studies of mind* (pp. 37–55). Cambridge, UK: Cambridge University Press.

Index

Accommodation. *See* Piagetian theory
Active role of the child
  developmental changes in, 31–33
  in family processes, 57
  in guided participation, 97–98
  in intersubjectivity, 80, 82
  in joint attention, 88
  in Piagetian theory, 25, 142
  in planning, 31–33, 178–179, 205
  in problem solving, 142
  in shared remembering, 118–120
  in sibling interactions, 59
  in social interaction, 30–34, 68
  in social referencing, 94–97
  in sociocultural theory, 30–34, 46
  in Vygotskian theory, 35, 37
Activities
  children's participation in, 4–5, 30, 39–40,
    56–57, 91, 211
  neighborhood resources, 56–57
  planning, 175–176, 195–197
  prior experience with, 58
  socially organized, 61–62
  in sociocultural theory, 40, 214
Activity theory
  as a theory, 44, 47–54, 213
  basic premises of, 48
  goal-directed behavior, 48–49
  introduction in the West, 48
  limitations of, 53–54
  parents' goals and, 12
  relation to other theories, 46, 213
  role of cultural and social history, 49–51
  unit of analysis, 44, 48–49
Adult–child interaction
  effects of, 43–44, 46
  processes of, 4

See also Adult–child planning; Adult–child
    problem solving; Guided participation
Adult–child planning
  active role of child, 178–179
  age related changes, 183
  and children's later individual planning, 183–
    184
  benefits of, 205
  child compliance and, 202–204
  errand planning, 182–185, 200
  future-oriented talk, 180–182
  in early and middle childhood, 182–185
  in infancy and toddlerhood, 178–182
  intentionality and, 178–180
  shared social history, 202–204
  sharing task responsibility, 200–201
  strategy development and, 184, 204–205
  variation in, 184–185
  verbal interaction in, 184–185
  versus peer, 186–188, 192–193, 204–206
  zone of proximal development, 183–184
Adult–child problem solving
  active role of child, 142
  attachment and, 168–169
  characteristics of child, 164–166
  characteristics of dyad, 168–169
  characteristics of partner, 166–168
  child age and, 164
  concept development and, 144
  contingent responding, 146
  development and, 155
  encoding and, 149–150, 169
  feedback and, 151–152
  goals and subgoals, 149, 153–154
  in early childhood, 145–152
  in infancy, 141–143
  joint attention and, 141–142